ACUPRESSURE
— FOR —
COMMON AILMENTS

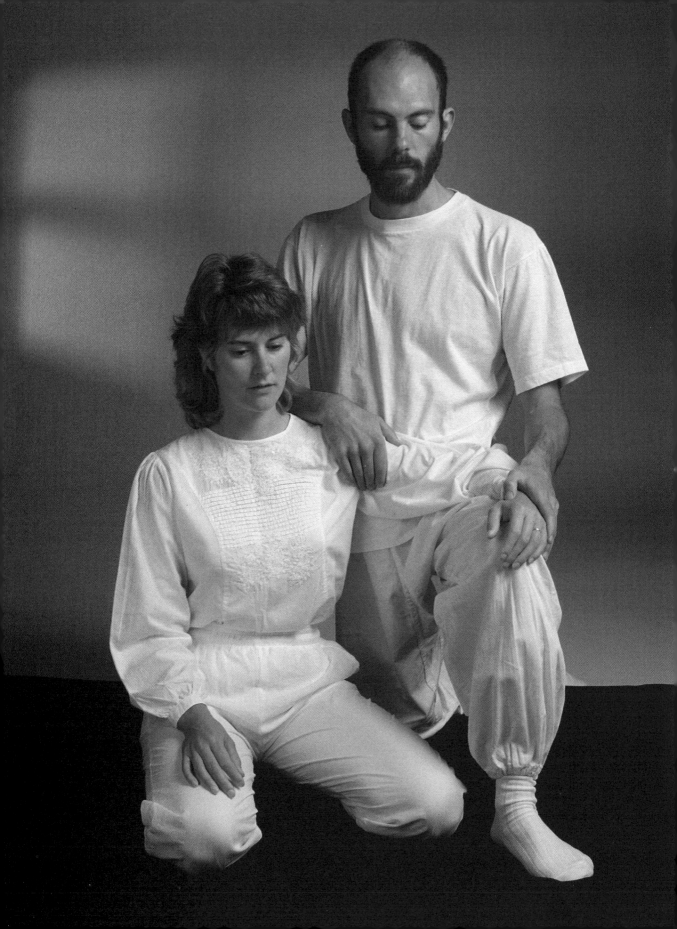

ACUPRESSURE
FOR
COMMON AILMENTS

Chris Jarmey

John Tindall

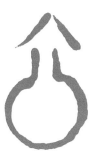

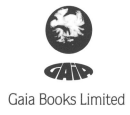

Gaia Books Limited

A GAIA ORIGINAL

Conceived by   Joss Pearson

Editorial   Eleanor Lines
Katherine Pate

Design   Dave Thorp

Photography   Fausto Dorelli

Illustration   Alison Champion

Art Direction   Patrick Nugent

® This is the Registered Trade Mark of
Gaia Books Limited.

First published in the United Kingdom in 1991 by
Gaia Books Limited   *and*
66 Charlotte Street,   20 High Street,
London W1P 1LR   Stroud, Glos GL5 1AS.

Typeset by Cambridge Photosetting Services, U.K.
Reproduction by Fotographics Ltd, Hong Kong
Printed and bound by Mateu Cromo, Spain

British Library Cataloguing in Publication Data
Jarmey, Chris
    Acupressure for common ailments.
    1. Acupressure
    I. Title   II. Tindall, John
    615.822

    ISBN 1-85675-015-9
    10 9 8 7 6

Caution
The techniques, ideas, and suggestions in this book are not
intended as a substitute for proper medical advice. Any
application of the techniques, ideas, and suggestions in this
book is at the reader's sole discretion and risk.

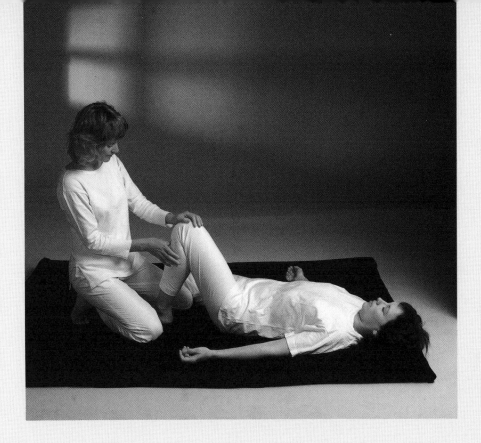

HOW TO USE THIS BOOK

Acupressure for Common Ailments is a manual, providing clear and concise directions for the use of thumb and finger pressure for relief of the symptoms of common ailments. It is for interested novices as well as students of acupressure, shiatsu, and massage. Part One outlines the concepts of Oriental medicine, explains how and why acupressure is such an effective therapy, and directs you in the simple techniques of acupressure. Part Two, arranged by ailment, gives clear instructions on which points to treat.

NB Capitalization of common terms such as Energy in this book denotes the Oriental rather than Western meaning (see p. 14).

A note on clothing

Wear loose cotton clothing for both giving and receiving acupressure, to allow maximum freedom of movement. Natural fibres are preferable to synthetics, which interfere with the flow of Energy in the Channels. Thin cotton is ideal: it allows the giver to focus on the recipient's body Energy rather than his/her skin or clothing. The illustrations in this book were modelled with minimum clothing in order to show the pressure points as clearly as possible.

A caution

Always consult a doctor if you are in doubt about a medical condition, and observe the cautions given in the treatment plans.

Contents

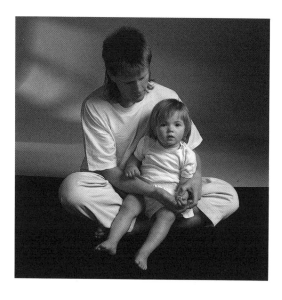

Introduction   8

Part one

ORIENTAL MEDICINE – The basic concepts   13
   Causes of disease   18
   The Channels and pressure points   20
   Major acupressure points   24
   Preparing to treat   28
   Herbs and oils   30
   Channel-opening techniques   32

Part two

TREATING COMMON AILMENTS   37
   General vitality   38
   Nervous system   40
   Immune system   46

Respiration   50
Digestion   57
Elimination   61
Circulation   64
Reproductive system   66
Bones and joints   73
Muscles   80
Sense organs   86

Summary of points   89

Index   93

Acknowledgements   95

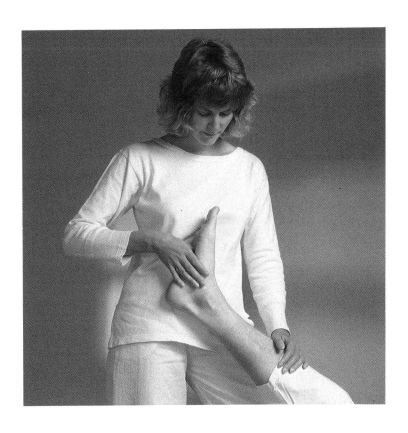

Introduction

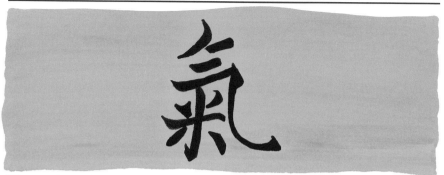

The ancient therapy known as acupressure has evolved from the same roots as the Oriental arts of shiatsu and acupuncture. The Oriental medical view describes how the body works in terms of its Energy, or Qi, rather than in the mechanical terms we are more familiar with in the West. Oriental therapies work by treating imbalances in the level and flow of our bodies' Energy. Acupressure uses finger pressure on the acupuncture points to manipulate the Energy imbalances. It may be used as part of a shiatsu treatment. However, used on its own, it is an effective therapy for home treatment. This book shows you how to practise acupressure at home to help your friends and family.

This vital Energy, known as Qi, is what keeps our bodies functioning and keeps us active. The main source of Qi is Universal Qi, which is all around us and provides the life force of all living things. Other sources of Qi include the air we breathe and the food we eat.

To an Oriental medicine practitioner, the quality of our Qi depends on the state of balance between our mental/emotional, physical, and spiritual aspects. When these aspects are in step with each other, we enjoy good health. But an imbalance in any one of them, whether as a result of an emotional trauma or of a virus, will alter our equilibrium and call for our bodies to readjust. Constant readjustment taxes our Qi, and from time to time we will not be able to respond sufficiently well to restore the harmony between our minds, our bodies, and our emotions, resulting in illness.

How acupressure works

The treatment system known as acupressure involves working on a recipient's Qi by pressing the fingers and thumbs on specific points that are located along Channels (also known as Meridians) of Qi (see pp. 22-23). These pressure points are the places where the Channels come near to the body's surface, making it possible to influence the Qi there. By manipulating the points you can either strengthen, disperse, or calm the Qi, helping it to flow smoothly in the body and to bring a harmonious relationship between body and mind, relieving any symptoms.

Knowledge of the Channels and pressure points has arisen from thousands of years of medical practice in China and more recently in Japan. Each of the major Channels is connected to a specific organ from which it takes its name: for example, Large Intestine Channel or Lung Channel. The health of the organs depends on the smooth flow of Qi in the Channels, and this can be regulated by acupressure. These basic concepts are explained in more detail in Part One.

Using acupressure for common ailments

Oriental medicine always seeks the underlying cause of disease, concentrating on the level and flow of Qi in the body. An experienced practitioner will develop a "treatment plan" tailored to the needs of the individual patient. To enable you to begin to treat your friends, Part Two describes treatment plans that take the most likely causes of each ailment into account. They give a quick-formula approach that will allow you to treat an ailing friend quickly and safely. If you can recognize the symptoms of an ailment in the very early stages, acupressure can often prevent its further development, or reduce its severity.

Although this book presents acupressure techniques for treating many of the most widely encountered ailments, **it is not intended to replace professional health care.** For serious diseases, such as AIDS, cancer, and heart disease, and for other serious health problems, such as obesity, high blood pressure, diabetes, allergies, alcoholism, and drug abuse, you should advise your friend to consult a skilled therapist or doctor who can determine a patient's individual needs. But you can also help to relieve some of the discomforts associated with any of these more serious ailments yourself, by following the treatment plan for stimulating the immune system (p. 48), and the plans for general vitality (p. 38), and anxiety and worry (p. 42), all of which will be beneficial. For people with heart or blood pressure problems, you can in addition use the techniques given on page 64, to improve the circulation.

Getting started

Acupressure is a very versatile form of treatment that can be given whenever and wherever it is convenient. You can use the techniques anywhere, from the office to outside in the garden, since it is not necessary to remove the recipient's clothing. The only equipment required is a pair of hands! Treatment is traditionally and most easily given with the recipient lying on a 'futon' or cotton mattress on the floor, but a folded blanket or towels are suitable alternatives.

When giving acupressure, both you and the recipient should wear loose, comfortable clothing, in order to have freedom of movement for the treatment. In this book the treatments have been illustrated with the recipients wearing very little clothing, in order to show the positions of the pressure points clearly. But in practice it is better for the recipient to wear a thin layer of clothing, for without it, your attention may be

restricted to the feel and texture of the skin, rather than to the subtle flow of Qi in the Channels. Ideally clothing should be made of thin cotton fabric, as synthetic fibres tend to affect the flow of Qi within the Channels. An experienced practitioner can feel the quality of a recipient's Qi beneath the surface of the skin.

How to give treatment

When giving acupressure, try to relax and keep your mind focused on what you are doing, allowing Universal Qi to flow into you and to replenish the Qi you are giving out. Think of yourself as an instrument for a more universal healing process. Be aware of your breathing: during treatment especially it should be deep and relaxed. Your own Qi helps to strengthen the weakened Qi of the person you are treating, so it is important that your Qi and vitality are stronger than that of your recipient. You should work to maintain your own Qi by eating fresh, nutritious food.

Before starting a treatment, you might like to use the "Channel-opening" techniques described in Part One. The different techniques for applying pressure to the pressure points are explained in *Preparing to treat*

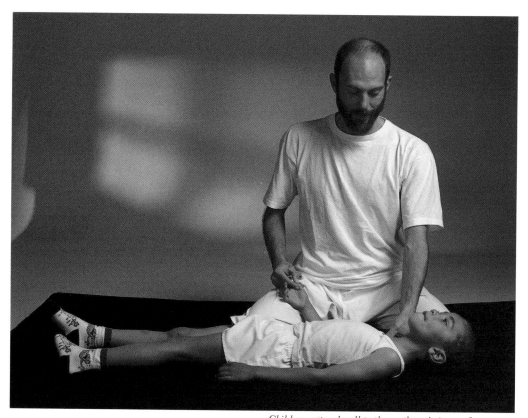

Children respond well to the gentle techniques of acupressure.

(p. 29). You can treat the pressure points on either side of the body (see pp. 22-23). Begin with the point nearest the affected part. To complement your acupressure treatment, try also using the herbs and oils recommended in each of the treatment plans in Part Two. Full instructions are given on pages 30-31.

Self-treatment with acupressure is also possible. You should concentrate on visualizing Universal Qi being channelled through your body to augment your own Qi as you apply pressure. Treating yourself, however, cannot be as effective as receiving acupressure from a practitioner who projects strong Qi. Also, you will not be able to reach some of your own pressure points – for example, those on your upper back. In this case, you can try lying on a golf ball to apply pressure to the points.

Babies and children benefit enormously from acupressure. Young children may find it difficult to sit still, so make sure they are comfortable and try treating them when they are sleepy. Consult a qualified practitioner before giving herbs and oils to children.

Emotional and physical reactions to treatment

Since acupressure is a gentle form of therapy, it is rare to have any negative emotional or physical reactions to the treatment. However, the recipient may experience some slight reaction if you are reaching the deep-rooted cause of a chronic (long-term) complaint. If Qi is strengthened and moves suddenly after a long period of stagnation, it can move accumulated toxins with it. The body will try to rid itself of these toxins, and this can cause a range of physical symptoms, such as headaches or skin rashes. There may also be emotional reactions, resulting in the recipient feeling upset or melancholic, for example. These symptoms should be short-lived, however, and you can continue with the treatment, provided the recipient is also willing.

When not to use acupressure

Acupressure is very safe. If by any chance you accidentally apply pressure to the wrong pressure points, the energy will rebalance itself in a day or two, with no ill-effects. There are, however, certain conditions where treatment is contra-indicated. You should not apply pressure to an open wound, or to a place where there is inflammation or swelling. Avoid any areas of scar tissue, boils, blisters, rashes, or varicose veins. If possible, treat the corresponding point on the opposite side of the body. For example, if the recipient has a varicose vein on the inner side of the left leg (requiring treatment to Spleen 6), you may help it by treating the same point on the other leg.

In addition, there are two pressure points that you should not use on people with high or low blood pressure, and three others that you should avoid during pregnancy, as they can cause miscarriage (see pp. 88–90). A "caution" is given with these points each time they occur, to remind you.

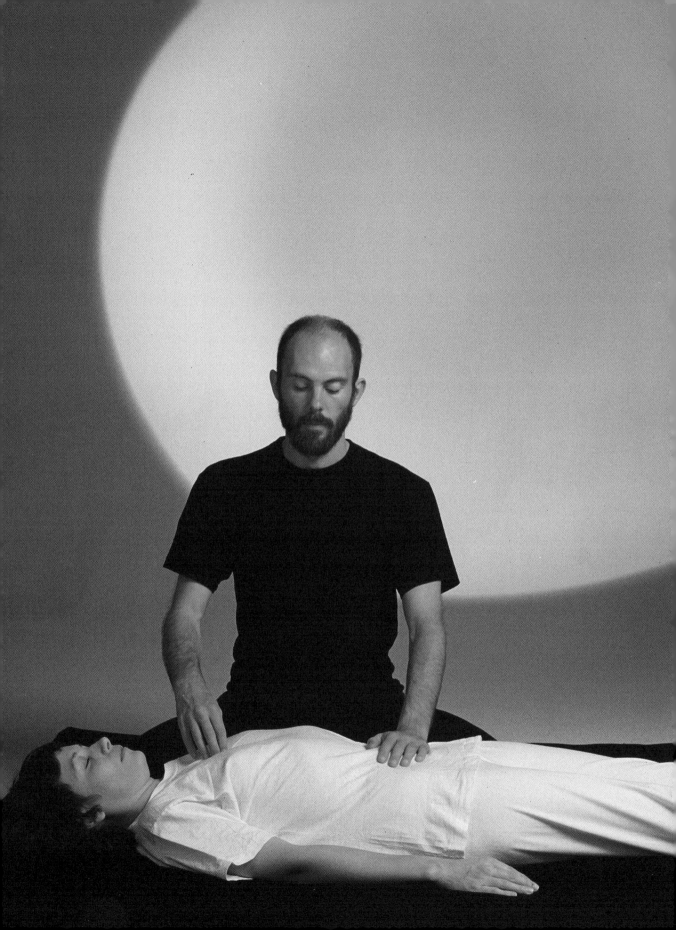

Part one

ORIENTAL MEDICINE
THE BASIC CONCEPTS

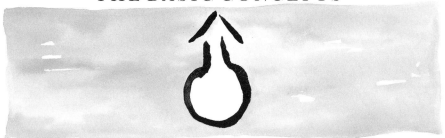

Understanding why acupressure works requires an appreciation of the Chinese system of diagnosis and treatment, where the fundamental approach to medicine bears little resemblance to that in the West.

Oriental medicine and Western medicine are able to treat the same conditions, but practitioners from East and West diagnose an ailment in completely different ways. Western doctors try to isolate an agent such as a virus, seen as the direct cause of an ailment, and then aim to eradicate it. Where the cause is not so simple or clear, as with the degenerative diseases, for example, Western medicine will tackle only the symptoms. Oriental practitioners, by contrast, look for a complete picture of their patient. This is known as the "pattern of disharmony". This pattern is built up by close observation of the patient's complexion, general demeanour, colour of urine, voice quality, and so on (see p. 21). The patient also answers a series of questions, including how external influences such as eating, touch, or heat affect the symptoms. A total picture is produced, and the diagnosis then made. The information in this book will enable you to understand how this is done. It takes many years to master the art of diagnosis, but you can offer helpful treatment by looking up a symptom, such as headache, asthma, or indigestion (see Part Two, *Treating common ailments*), and following the suggested treatment plan. These treatments are designed to cover the most likely causes of the symptoms.

The most fundamental concept of Oriental medicine is that your body, mind, and spirit are all interdependent. They affect one another at all levels: an ailment of the mind will be reflected in the body; similarly, any physical symptoms must affect the emotions and the psyche. The Oriental doctor does not see a physical ailment in isolation, but as a reflection of disharmony within your whole being. In addition to treating you, the doctor would also recommend that you consider the way you live, and evaluate your own weaknesses that are disrupting your body's equilibrium. Thus acupressure treatment helps to restore the harmony of body, mind, and spirit.

The functions of the organs

This holistic approach in Oriental medicine is also seen in the wide interpretation given to the functions of the organs. For example, the anatomical organ "kidney" referred to in Oriental medicine has a much broader meaning than in Western medicine. An Oriental doctor takes into account the work of the kidney not only in water metabolism, but also in providing a link between sources of energy and growth, the bones and brain, willpower and memory. For this reason, the Oriental medical concept will be presented with an initial capital letter – Kidney – to differentiate it from the strict anatomical meaning used by Western doctors. Similarly, an initial capital letter for other organs indicates a wider connotation. You will find other terms throughout this book that also take an initial capital letter. Oriental medicine interprets these all more widely than in the West.

The importance of Energy

The flow of vital Energy is essential to our health and fundamental to the practice of acupressure. The Chinese call this Energy "Qi", or "Chi". Qi supplies our Organs, Blood, and other Body Fluids, as well as the Mind. It is also responsible for the life processes, from conception through birth and growth, until death. When your body is in good health, your Qi flows abundantly and smoothly. If your Qi becomes deficient or blocked in any way, disease may result. Acupressure can unblock congested Qi, strengthen weak Qi, and calm overactive Qi.

The Channels

According to Oriental theory Qi circulates along Channels close to the body's surface. Many Channels have been identified, 12 of which link points that are connected to a particular Organ in the body. The Channels are named after the Organ to which they are linked – Liver Channel, Gall Bladder Channel, Large Intestine Channel, and so on. Located along these Channels are the specific points, known as pressure points, where you can most easily manipulate Qi using acupressure (see p. 20). By applying pressure to these points you can unblock, strengthen, or calm the flow of Qi, depending on the technique used (see p. 29). For example, there is a pressure point located four finger widths below your kneecap, outside the tibia (or shin bone), known as Stomach 36, on the Channel related to your Stomach. Correct pressure on this point will strengthen your Stomach and Spleen and aid digestion.

Yin and Yang

Good health depends on the smooth flow of Qi along the Channels, and this in turn requires the body and mind to be in harmony. A balance in all the aspects of your personality and of your physical body will provide this harmony. The Chinese use the idea of Yin and Yang to express this idea of balance. Yin originally meant the shady side of a slope. It is

associated with such qualities as cold, rest, responsiveness, passivity, darkness, interiority, downwardness, inwardness, decrease, and femininity. Yang, by contrast, originally referred to the sunny side of a slope. It implies brightness, and is associated with qualities such as heat, stimulation, movement, activity, excitement, vigour, light, exteriority, upwardness, outwardness, increase, and masculinity. Yin and Yang are complementary opposites (see p. 17). Everything in the universe has both Yin and Yang qualities – nothing is completely one or the other. It is the interaction between these two opposite forces that creates Qi. If your body Energy is well balanced your Qi will have both Yin and Yang aspects. If the balance of Yin and Yang qualities in any aspect of your mind or body is disrupted, then so too will be the Qi in your body, and ill health may result.

Treatment plan

The skilled practitioner diagnoses the Yin and Yang imbalances from the pattern of disharmony and then decides on the treatment plan. First, by recognizing the origin of an ailment in a particular Organ of the body, the practitioner can establish which Channel and points to work on. The summary of correspondences chart on page 21 gives more details of the links between the Organs and the Channels. Second, the practitioner decides on the type of acupressure technique to be used. This depends on whether Qi is blocked, deficient, or in excess. Deficient Qi must be tonified, blocked Qi dispersed, and overactive Qi calmed. When Qi becomes blocked, overactive, or deficient, the symptoms and their link with a particular Organ or part of the body will be recognizable to the trained eye. For example, lethargy is a symptom of a Qi deficiency in the whole body, whereas incontinence or oedema would be the result of a Kidney Qi deficiency. If Kidney Qi were not deficient, but instead blocked or overactive, different symptoms would result. The techniques for tonifying, dispersing, and calming Qi are demonstrated on page 29 and each treatment in the book specifies which technique to use for each pressure point to be treated.

The skill of diagnosing ailments and making treatment plans takes years to master, but even as a beginner you can help restore wellbeing. Part Two, *Treating common ailments*, gives treatment plans for the most common causes of the conditions and ailments described.

Use this book wisely. *Do not try to take over a doctor's role – help where you can and seek medical advice where you cannot.*

Yin and Yang

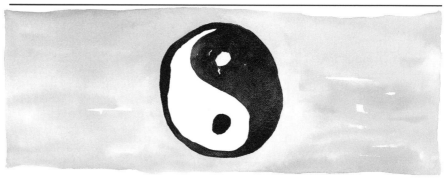

The formal origins of Oriental medicine lie in the philosophy known as Taoism, first developed by Lao Tzu after about 600BC. At the core of this philosophy is the belief that human beings are part of nature. This means that we experience the constant flow and change of nature, and it is this flow and change that is reality. Many of us try to create permanence in our lives and in the objects around us, but, because reality is in a state of flux, we should instead try to maintain a state of balance within this constant change. It is this balance that gives us a sense of harmony and wellbeing, and is the source of our health.

Chinese medical theory looks for a logic in the patterns of change, and the Yin Yang theory was developed to explain these patterns. The terms Yin and Yang are used to describe the qualities of all things, and their relationship to each other and the universe. Everything contains Yin and Yang elements: Yin and Yang are opposite and complementary.

The balance of Yin Qi and Yang Qi in your body is crucial to your health. Four variations in the Yin Yang balance of Qi are common:

1. Normal balance and quantity of Yin and Yang Qi, which represents health.

2. Normal Yin Qi, but excess Yang Qi, which creates Heat and overactivity.

3. Normal Yang Qi, but deficient Yin Qi, creating Heat (especially at night) and a lack of vitality.

4. Normal Yin Qi, but deficient Yang Qi, creating lethargy, chilliness and poor circulation.

The chart opposite illustrates how the possible imbalances (numbers 2-4 above) may affect your health. The acupressure techniques of calming, tonifying, and dispersing are described on page 29.

From the chart opposite you will see that deficiencies of Yang lead to Yin-type symptoms; deficiencies in Yin will produce Yang-type symptoms. Nothing can be wholly Yin or Yang because there are no fixed extremes in nature. The qualities of Yin and Yang are always relative: warm water, for example, is more Yang than ice, but more Yin than steam. Some of these qualities are outlined in the table opposite.

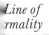

*Line of
rmality*

YIN **YANG**

Excess Yang (Yin normal)
Overall Qi is in excess. This results in Heat and overactivity, a full, flushed, red face, and often an overbearing personality.

A dispersing or calming treatment is required, because Qi is in excess and possibly blocked or overactive.

YIN **YANG**

Deficient Yin (Yang normal)
Overall Qi is lacking. This results in "empty" Heat, because the cooling quality of Yin is absent. Symptoms similar to excess Yang appear, such as insomnia, dry mouth, and nervous excitability.

Pressure points and Channels require tonification, because overall Qi is deficient.

YIN **YANG**

Deficient Yang (Yin normal)
Overall Qi is lacking. This results in chilliness because the warming quality of Yang is absent. Symptoms include tiredness and poor circulation. This often leads to excessive Damp or Phlegm in the body, which may result in catarrh, or even cysts or tumours.

Pressure points and Channels require tonification, because overall Qi is deficient, and also warming because Yang is deficient.

Note *The symptoms of excess Yin Qi with normal Yang Qi are similar to those of excess Yang Qi, but this condition is extremely rare.*

General correspondences of Yin and Yang

YIN	YANG
Shade	Brightness
Female	Male
Moon	Sun
Rest	Activity
Material	Immaterial
Contraction	Expansion
Soft	Hard

Yin and Yang manifestations in the body

YIN	YANG
Front	Back
Organ's substance	Energy supplying organs
Interior Organs	Exterior skin, muscles
Blood, Body Fluids	Qi
Moist	Dry
Slow	Rapid
Cold	Hot
Sinking	Rising

Yin and Yang symptoms

YIN	YANG
Chronic disease	Acute disease
Gradual onset	Rapid onset
Pale face	Red face
Not thirsty	Thirsty
Loose stools	Constipation
Cold	Heat
Sleepiness	Restlessness, insomnia

The treatments recommended in this book take into account the balance of Yin and Yang, and use one of the four following strategies:
1. Tonify Yang Qi
2. Tonify Yin Qi
3. Disperse, calm, or eliminate excess Yang Qi
4. Disperse, calm, or eliminate excess Yin Qi (rare)

The causes of disease

For you to get the most out of this book, it will help if you understand how traditional Oriental medicine views the causes of disease. Oriental practitioners do not treat the symptoms of a disease, they look for the underlying causes of it, which are always expressed as disruption of Qi, Yin, and Yang in various parts of the body.

According to Oriental medicine the causes of disease fall into three categories: internal (the emotions); external (the weather), and other causes such as germs or poisons, trauma, diet, and the effects of drugs.

The diseases resulting from emotional causes can be very deep-rooted and are the most difficult to treat. The effects of these causes are described below.

The main external factor – weather – is usually only disabling if your resistance is already low. Nowadays, environmental pollution is probably as important a cause of disease as the weather. Some of the specific effects of weather on the body are described opposite.

Ailments caused by germs, diet, and so on are the most easily treated. But the symptoms, if ignored, can produce effects as far-reaching as those due to the weather or emotions.

Recognizing the cause of a symptom will enable you to offer positive advice to support your treatment. Acupressure will help to bring the Yin and Yang elements back into harmony, and restore the circulation of Qi.

EMOTIONS

Each of the emotions affects the harmony of particular Organs. It is natural to feel sadness, anger, or joy when the occasion demands it, but it is harmful if an emotion such as anger is harboured for years. Since fighting these disturbances creates even more conflict, the Oriental way is to observe them with awareness and allow them to be. Through meditation they will naturally quieten and abate.

Joy
Joyful emotions are fundamentally strengthening for the body and mind. However, excessive excitement can lead to over-stimulation of the Heart, causing mental restlessness, palpitations, insomnia, and mouth or tongue ulcers.

Fear
Fear can mean anything from terror to a lack of self-confidence. It diminishes the Energy of the Kidneys, especially the cooling Yin aspect, and may give rise to palpitations, night sweating, and a dry mouth and throat; plus bedwetting in children.

Anger
Emotions from resentment to animosity affect the Liver Energy. Excessive or prolonged anger causes Qi to rise, resulting in tinnitus, thirst, dizziness, or vomiting, but most commonly, headaches. It can also cause Liver Energy to interfere with the Spleen's digestive function, causing diarrhoea, especially if angry rows occur at mealtimes. Repressed anger or resentment may lead to chronic depression.

Sadness and grief

These cause a deficiency of Lung Energy, which impairs the Lung's ability to take in and distribute Qi through the body and mind. They deplete Qi generally and particularly interfere with the Heart. They can lead to tiredness, breathlessness, depression, and crying. In women, menstruation can cease, because Blood becomes deficient due to the effect of sadness on the Heart.

Overthinking and worry

Excessive mental work or study depletes Spleen Energy, thus interfering with digestion and causing tiredness, loose stools, and lack of appetite. Worry also interferes with the Lungs, resulting in breathlessness, anxiety, and stiffness in the neck and shoulders.

Mental shock

This depletes Heart Qi suddenly, often leading to breathlessness and palpitations. Shock can also interfere with the harmony of the Mind, which is linked with the Heart, causing insomnia. Shock also depletes the Energy of the Kidney, especially the cooling Yin aspect, and can lead to dizziness, night sweating, or tinnitus.

WEATHER

Extremes of weather can affect people when their resistance is low. The symptoms are usually similar in nature to the weather that caused them.

Wind

Symptoms caused by wind predominantly affect the head and may come on suddenly and change rapidly, like gusts of wind. Common symptoms are stiff neck, runny nose, sneezing, coughing, and aversion to cold. Wind can directly affect the Channels, particularly the Liver Channel, causing stiff and painful joints, wandering pains, and migraines.

Cold

The body tissues contract in cold weather, obstructing Blood circulation and resulting in stiffness, chilliness, and pain, most frequently in the limbs, shoulders, and lower back. Cold in the stomach causes vomiting after eating; in the intestines it causes abdominal pain and diarrhoea, and in the uterus, acute painful menstruation. Cold is always implicated when there are thin, clear, watery, and cool discharges from the body.

Damp

This type of weather produces sticky, heavy symptoms beginning in the legs and moving upward. It may cause vaginal discharges if it reaches the female genital system; loose stools if it reaches the intestines; frequent, burning, and difficult urination if it settles in the bladder; and swollen, aching joints if it gets into the Channels. Damp produces these symptoms because it weakens the Spleen's function of transforming food into body tissues, leading to an accumu-lation of phlegm and fluids.

Dryness

Dry lips, mouth, tongue, throat, dry stools, and scanty urination, are all due to drying of the body fluids. Heat causes thirst, sweating, headaches, and an aversion to heat. In extreme cases it can cause delirium, slurred speech, and mental restlessness or even unconsciousness.

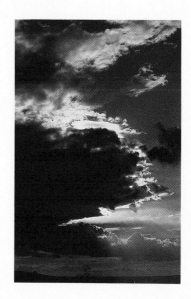

The Channels and pressure points

The Channels, also known as Meridians, are the pathways through the body along which Qi flows. There are 12 major Channels, each linked to the function of a particular Organ, plus two extra Channels that run up the torso and head on the front and back (see pp. 22-23). The pathways run in a circuitous route through and around the body. They rise at intervals toward the surface, and dip deeper into the body, leading to the Organs. The Channels also have wider connections that create a network throughout the body, and they are each paired with another Channel. One of the pair has Yin characteristics; the other, Yang (see pp. 16-17). The chart opposite summarizes the main functions of the Organs and presents the Organs and Channels in their pairs, showing which are Yin and which are Yang.

Pressure points

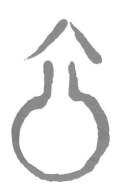

The pressure points, or acupoints, are the gateways to the Channels. Here the Qi in a Channel comes close to the skin and can be manipulated using acupressure. The locations of the pressure points used in this book are illustrated on pages 22-23 and described in the treatment plans in Part Two, and in the *Summary of points* (pp. 89-91).

The shape of these pressure points (or "tsubos", as they are also known), should not be thought of in physical terms: it can only be described in terms of Energy. Imagine them shaped like a vase, with a neck and mouth narrower than the base. The Japanese character for a pressure point (left) illustrates this shape.

The techniques for applying pressure to the pressure points, to tonify, disperse, or calm the Qi in the Channels, are described on page 29.

The table lists the five elements – the fundamental components of the Universe – that govern the Channels (according to Oriental thinking). It also gives some of the emotional and physical characteristics that are traditionally associated with the Channels and the type of weather most damaging to each Organ and Channel.

While it would be rare to find someone corresponding to the archetypal groups of characteristics shown, you can still see tendencies in people. Consider a person's attitude to a colour (a great love or strong aversion); any tendency to display a particular emotion, or a tendency to problems in a sense organ (for example, a poor sense of smell).

If three or more characteristic problems correspond to one Channel, it suggests an imbalance in that Channel. For example, a person who feels worse in very dry weather, is often sad, whose voice has a weeping quality, and who has skin problems, may benefit from acupressure on the Lung or Large Intestine Channels.

A skilled practitioner considers all these correspondences in completing the patient's "pattern of disharmony" (see p. 13). These connections have been used in compiling the treatment plans in Part Two, Treating common ailments.

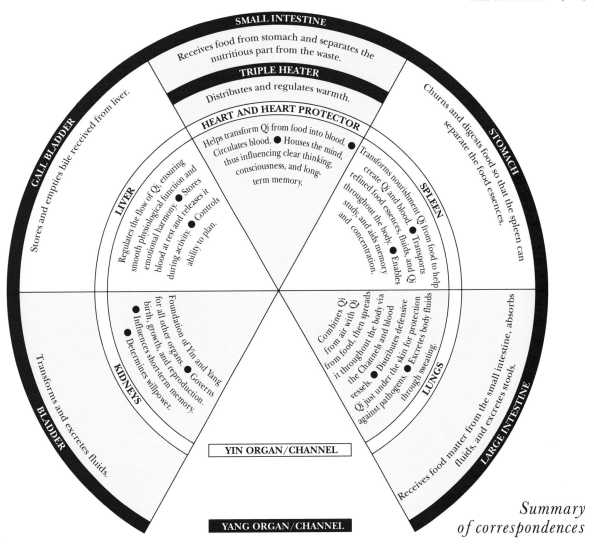

Summary of correspondences

| | Lu | Sp | H & HP | Liv | K |
	LI	**St**	**SI & TH**	**GB**	**B**
Element	Metal	Earth	Fire	Wood	Water
Season	Autumn	Late Summer	Summer	Spring	Winter
Colour	White	Yellow	Red	Green	Black
Sense Organ	Nose	Mouth	Tongue	Eyes	Ears
Tissue	Skin	Muscles	Blood Vessels	Ligaments	Bones
Voice quality	Weeping	Singing	Laughing	Shouting	Groaning
Emotion	Sadness	Pensiveness	Joy	Anger	Fear
Body odour	Rotten	Fragrant	Burning	Rancid	Putrid
Weather	Dryness	Damp	Heat	Wind	Cold

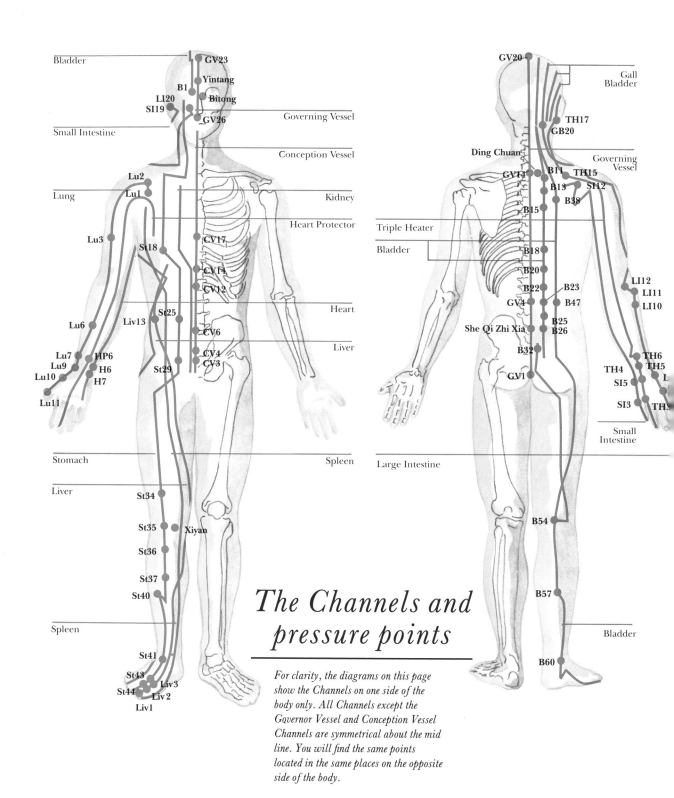

Bladder

GV23

Yintang

B1

Bitong

LI20

SI19

GV26

Governing Vessel

Small Intestine

Conception Vessel

Lu2

Lu1

Lung

Kidney

Lu3

St18

CV17

Heart Protector

CV14

CV12

Lu6

Liv13

St25

Heart

Lu7

Lu9

HP6

H6

H7

CV6

CV4

CV3

Liver

Lu10

Lu11

St29

Stomach

Spleen

Liver

St34

St35

Xiyan

St36

St37

St40

Spleen

St41

St43

St44

Liv3

Liv2

Liv1

GV20

Gall Bladder

TH17

GB20

Ding Chuan

Governing Vessel

GV14

B11

TH15

B13

SI12

B38

B15

Triple Heater

Bladder

B18

B20

B22

B23

GV4

B47

She Qi Zhi Xia

B25

B26

B32

GV1

LI12

LI11

LI10

TH6

TH5

TH4

L

SI5

SI3

TH3

Small Intestine

Large Intestine

B54

B57

Bladder

B60

The Channels and pressure points

For clarity, the diagrams on this page show the Channels on one side of the body only. All Channels except the Governor Vessel and Conception Vessel Channels are symmetrical about the mid line. You will find the same points located in the same places on the opposite side of the body.

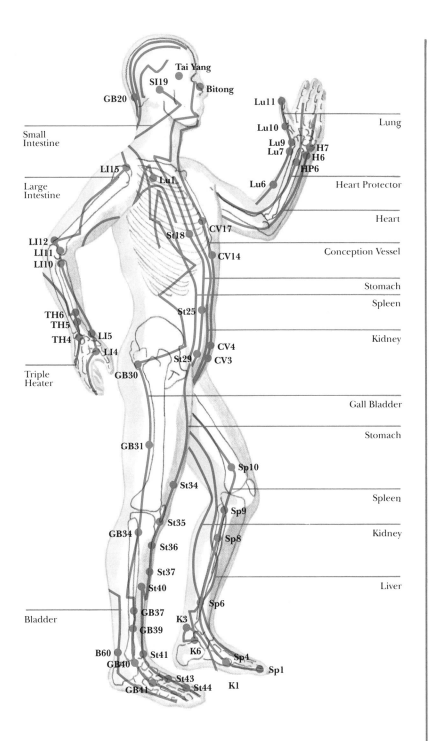

Tai Yang
SI19
Bitong
GB20
Lu11
Lung
Small
Intestine
Lu10
Lu9
Lu7
H7
H6
Large
Intestine
LI15
HP6
Lu1
Lu6
Heart Protector
Heart
St18
CV17
LI12
LI11
LI10
CV14
Conception Vessel
Stomach
Spleen
St25
Kidney
TH6
TH5
TH4
LI5
LI4
CV4
CV3
St29
Triple
Heater
GB30
Gall Bladder
Stomach
GB31
Sp10
St34
Spleen
Sp9
St35
Kidney
GB34
Sp8
St36
St37
St40
Liver
Sp6
GB37
K3
Bladder
GB39
B60
Sp4
GB40
St41
K6
Sp1
St43
K1
GB41
St44

Numbering the points

Each Channel is either more Yin or more Yang (see p. 21). The numbering of points on the Yin Channels starts from the feet and works upward, since Yin Energy comes from the earth. The points on the Yang Channels are numbered from the head downward, since Yang Energy comes from the sun.

Each Channel has a wider network of connections with other Channels. The treatments in Part Two take account of this network and recommend treating the points that bring most benefit because of their internal connections within the Channel network.

Location of points

To locate each acupressure point, first read the description of how to find it on the treatment plan. Then use the illustrations on pages 24-27 to build up a clearer idea of the bone structure, and the Summary on pages 88-91, with its anatomical illustrations, to become familiar with the skeleton as a whole.

Horary rhythm

The order of the Channels in the Key represents the order in which Qi is thought to flow through the Channels during a 24-hour cycle. Qi flows most strongly through the Lung Channel between 3am and 5am, and during the course of the day flows for two-hour periods in each Channel in turn, surging through them in the order shown.

Key	**Lu**	Lung
	LI	Large Intestine
	St	Stomach
	Sp	Spleen
	H	Heart
	SI	Small Intestine
	B	Bladder
	K	Kidney
	HP	Heart Protector
	TH	Triple Heater
	GB	Gall Bladder
	Liv	Liver
	CV	Conception Vessel
	GV	Governing Vessel

Major acupressure points

There are more than 660 pressure points, of which 365 are located on the major Channels illustrated on pages 22-23. You will find 97 of these points demonstrated in Part Two, *Treating common ailments*. The 12 pressure points shown on the following four pages, however, are the most commonly used in the book. They have very strong and far-reaching connections within the Channel network, which makes them particularly powerful. Therefore pressure applied to these points has long-lasting effects. How to apply pressure is described on page 29.

To help you locate the major pressure points, the illustrations below show the positions of the underlying bone structures. If you use these illustrations in conjunction with those of the major Channels (pp. 22-23), you should find it easy to feel your way into the major pressure points.
Caution Never use LI4 and Sp6 during pregnancy. They can cause miscarriage.

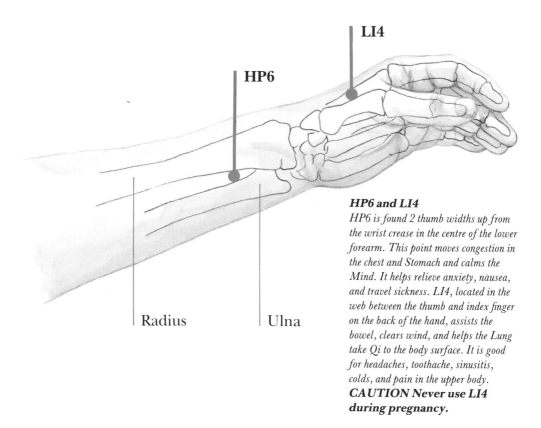

LI4

HP6

Radius Ulna

HP6 and LI4
HP6 is found 2 thumb widths up from the wrist crease in the centre of the lower forearm. This point moves congestion in the chest and Stomach and calms the Mind. It helps relieve anxiety, nausea, and travel sickness. LI4, located in the web between the thumb and index finger on the back of the hand, assists the bowel, clears wind, and helps the Lung take Qi to the body surface. It is good for headaches, toothache, sinusitis, colds, and pain in the upper body.
CAUTION Never use LI4 during pregnancy.

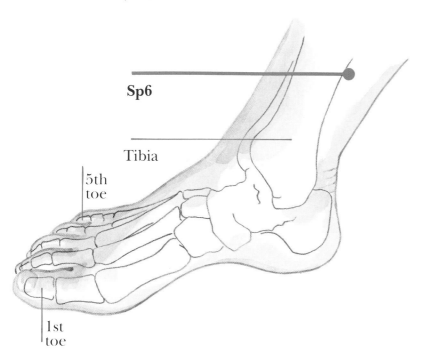

Sp6

Tibia

5th
toe

1st
toe

Sp6

Locate this point 4 finger widths above the inside ankle bone, just behind the tibia. This point connects with the Liver and Kidney Channels and strengthens the Yin Channels in the legs. It stimulates the circulation and production of Qi and Blood, and eliminates Dampness. It is good for poor digestion, period problems, sterility, difficult labour, insomnia, and anaemia.
CAUTION Never use Sp6 during pregnancy.

GB34, St36, and Liv3

GB34 is in the depression on the outer side of the lower leg below the knee joint, in front of and below the top of the fibula. This is a special point for all muscle and tendon problems. It calms the Liver and removes Damp Heat from the Liver and Gall Bladder Channels. St36 is 4 finger widths below the kneecap, outside the tibia. This point balances the Stomach and Spleen and regulates Qi and Blood. It is good for weak digestion, anxiety, headaches, pain in the legs, and poor circulation. Liv3 is in the furrow on the top of the foot between the first and second toes, where the bones merge. This point regulates the Liver to promote free-flowing Qi and Blood, and helps the Liver store Blood. It is used to treat migraines, period problems, digestive disorders, irritability, and insomnia.

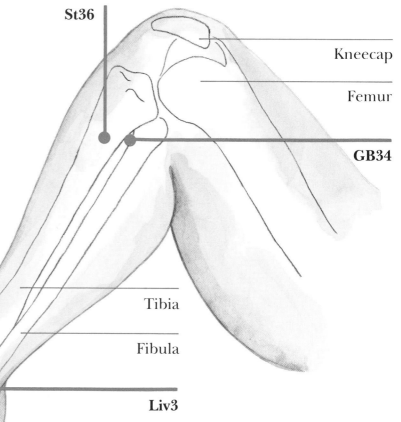

St36

Kneecap

Femur

GB34

Tibia

Fibula

Liv3

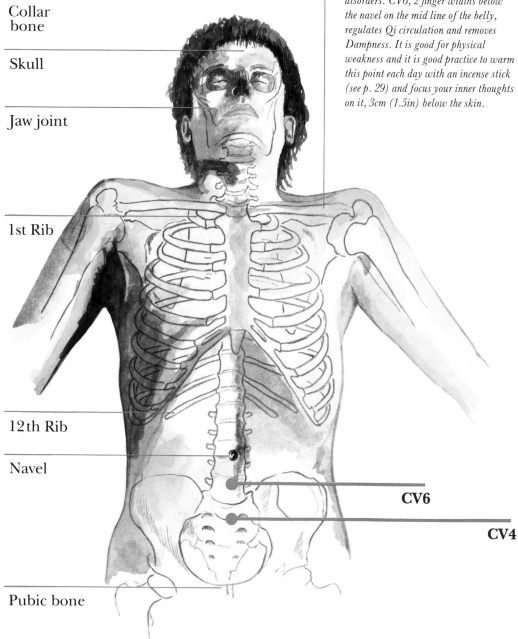

CV4 and CV6

CV4 is found 4 finger widths below the navel on the mid line of the belly. This point is also connected to the Liver, Spleen, Kidney, and Conception Vessel Channels. It invigorates the Blood and regulates menstruation. It is good for physical weakness and menstrual disorders. CV6, 2 finger widths below the navel on the mid line of the belly, regulates Qi circulation and removes Dampness. It is good for physical weakness and it is good practice to warm this point each day with an incense stick (see p. 29) and focus your inner thoughts on it, 3cm (1.5in) below the skin.

Collar bone

Skull

Jaw joint

1st Rib

12th Rib

Navel

CV6

CV4

Pubic bone

GB20

GB20 is found at the base of the skull in a hollow between the front and back neck muscles, behind the bony prominence behind the ear. This point clears Wind, calms Liver Qi, and disperses stagnant Qi in the head. It is used in treating headaches, colds, sinusitis, tension, and congestion in the head.

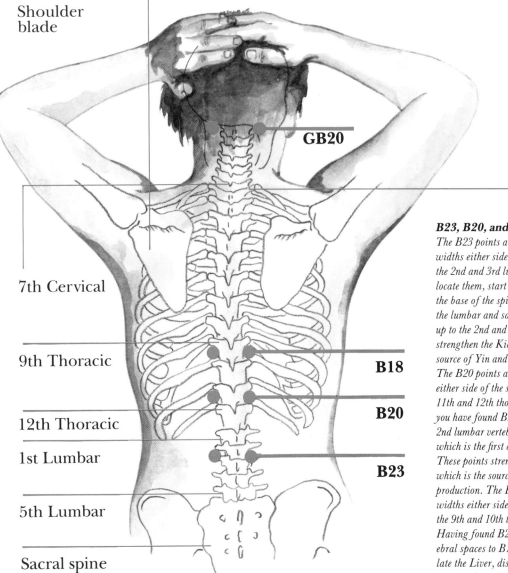

Shoulder blade

GB20

1st Thoracic

7th Cervical

B23, B20, and B18

The B23 points are found 2 finger widths either side of the spine, level with the 2nd and 3rd lumbar vertebrae. To locate them, start at the 5th lumbar at the base of the spine, at the junction of the lumbar and sacral spine, and count up to the 2nd and 3rd. These points strengthen the Kidneys, which are the source of Yin and Yang within the body. The B20 points are 2 finger widths either side of the spine, level with the 11th and 12th thoracic vertebrae. Once you have found B23, count up from the 2nd lumbar vertebra to the 12th thoracic, which is the first after the 1st lumbar. These points strengthen the Spleen, which is the source of Qi and Blood production. The B18 points are 2 finger widths either side of the spine, level with the 9th and 10th thoracic vertebrae. Having found B20, count up two vertebral spaces to B18. These points regulate the Liver, disperse stagnant Qi, and promote Blood circulation.

9th Thoracic

B18

B20

12th Thoracic

1st Lumbar

B23

5th Lumbar

Sacral spine

Preparing to treat

For effective acupressure treatment you and your recipient should both feel comfortable and relaxed. If you are tense, your recipient will feel it and become tense also.

To relax, concentrate on relaxing your belly, feeling its normal expansion and contraction as you breathe naturally. When your belly is relaxed, other tensions in your body disappear.

Both practitioner and recipient should wear loose clothing (see p. 5 and p. 9). The recipient should lie on a mat on the floor (see p. 9).

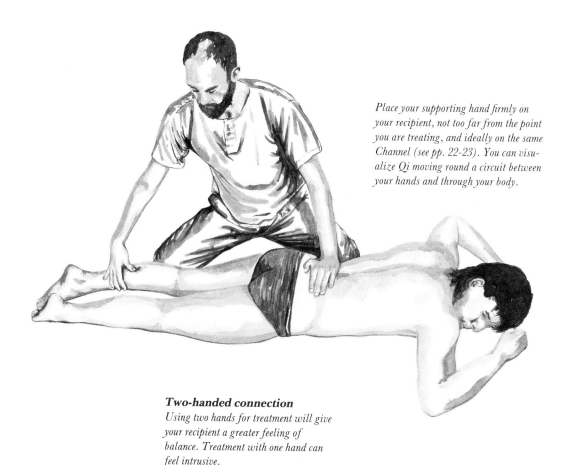

Place your supporting hand firmly on your recipient, not too far from the point you are treating, and ideally on the same Channel (see pp. 22-23). You can visualize Qi moving round a circuit between your hands and through your body.

Two-handed connection
Using two hands for treatment will give your recipient a greater feeling of balance. Treatment with one hand can feel intrusive.

As a general rule, try to keep several points of connection with your recipient, so the whole body is involved in your treatment, rather than just an isolated part. *For example, if you are kneeling beside the recipient, let your knee rest against him or her, provided you do not sacrifice your own comfort in doing so.*

TECHNIQUES FOR STIMULATING THE PRESSURE POINTS

There are three techniques for stimulating the pressure points – tonifying, dispersing, and calming – and these are described below. They all work to restore the equilibrium and strengthen the flow of Qi.

The general rule is: tonify weak Qi, disperse blocked or "stagnant" Qi, and calm overactive Qi. The treatment plans in Part Two tell you whether to tonify, calm, or disperse in each case. To find the pressure points, follow the instructions on each page of treatment. You can also refer to the *Summary of points* on pages 88-91 and the illustrations of the major points on pages 24-27.

Keep your arms relaxed and lean into the points to apply pressure. The points you treat may be sensitive, but the treatment should not be painful. Be guided by your recipient in how much pressure you apply.

You should treat the recommended points on the right and left sides of the body, to gain the full benefit of the treatment. For local complaints, for example, injuries to a specific part of the body, concentrate mainly on the affected side.

For chronic (long-term) conditions, treat the points every other day. For acute (short-term) conditions, treat them twice daily. Continue the treatments until the symptoms have disappeared.

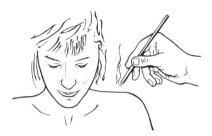

Warming with an incense stick
This is a tonifying technique. Hold the lighted incense stick 2cm (1in) from the pressure point, until the point feels pleasantly warm.

Tonifying and dispersing
To tonify Qi at a pressure point apply stationary pressure with your thumb or fingertip perpendicular to the point, and hold for about 2 minutes. As you do so, imagine the vase shape of the pressure point filling up with Qi (see p. 20). In some treatments tonifying with your elbow (see p. 49) or your thumbnail is recommended, to apply firmer pressure. To disperse Qi at a pressure point apply moving pressure with your thumb or fingertip in a circular motion, or "pumping" in and out of the point, for about 2 minutes. This encourages the smooth flow of Qi along the Channels.

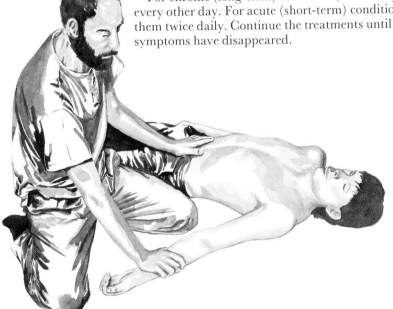

Calming
Use your palm to cover the point, or apply light moving pressure, for example, gentle stroking, for about 2 minutes.

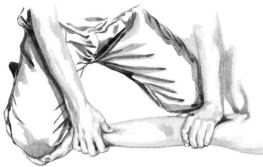

Herbs and oils

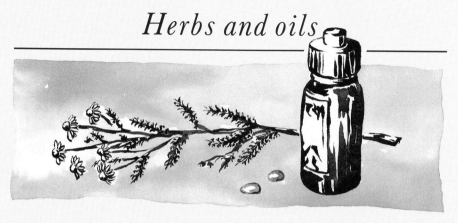

Simple preparations of herbs and oils can complement and augment your acupressure treatment. Traditional Chinese treatment often includes Chinese herbs. The herbs and oils recommended in this book are those used in Western herbalism and more readily available in the West. Specific herbs and oils are recommended for each treatment in Part Two of this book.

How to use

Both the herbs and oils can be used in baths and compresses. In addition, you can use herbs to make teas and poultices, and use oils in massage and inhalations. Instructions for their preparation are given opposite. Oils should not be taken internally. Compresses and poultices will help heal both external injuries and internal disorders: apply them to the affected area for periods of 15-20 minutes. Repeat this once daily for long-term conditions, or twice a day for short-term problems. Herb teas are particularly good for internal problems. All the herbs recommended in this book are safe to be drunk as teas. If a particular blend of herbs tastes unpleasant, try omitting some from the mixture. Herb or oil bath preparations, used for 15-20 minutes once or twice daily, can be helpful for both internal and external problems.

Where treatment with smelling salts is recommended, test the pungency of the mixture yourself first by smelling it. Old salts may become too pungent to hold close: hold them about 5cm (2in) away from the recipient.

Use herbs and oils with respect; their effects can be as powerful as any other medicine. Consult a qualified practitioner before giving herbs and oils to children. Additional cautions are given for the use of certain herbs and oils during pregnancy, as they can cause miscarriage. You will find the cautions clearly stated each time the herbs and oils are recommended for use.

Herbs

You can use dried herbs as teas, baths, compresses, or poultices. These treatments are all mild and are simple and safe to prepare. Where herbs are indicated, mix equal quantities of up to four of the herbs recommended.

Teas

For a mixture of leaves and flowers, use one teaspoon of mixed herbs per cup of boiling water. Cover and leave to infuse for 5-10 minutes. For roots or bark (crushed), boil one teaspoon per cup in water for 10-15 minutes. Strain the tea and add honey if desired. Never add milk or sugar. Drink one cup three times a day until the problem subsides.

Poultices

Mix powdered herbs in equal quantities, sufficient to cover the area to be treated, to a paste with hot water. Spread the paste on a sterile gauze, and place another gauze on top. Apply the poultice as hot as possible. When the poultice cools, repeat using more sterile gauzes.

Baths

Prepare the herbs as for tea and add the liquid to the bath water.

Compresses

Prepare the herbs as for tea. Dip a sterile gauze into the liquid, and apply it immediately. When the compress cools, repeat using another sterile gauze.

Oils

You can use essential oils for massage, inhalation, and in baths and compresses. Never use neat essential oils. They should always be diluted in a base oil for massage, or in water for baths, compresses and inhalations. For massage, mix 5-10 drops of each essential oil (up to 4 oils maximum) with 50ml (2fl oz) of base oil. Wheatgerm, avocado, sweet almond, and sunflower oils are good bases. The base oil should be 100% pure and unrefined. Mix only 50ml (2floz) at a time; the oil will keep for one to two months if stored in a dark, cold place.

Massage

Massage the oil into both the affected area and the pressure points suggested.

Baths

Add a maximum of 7 drops of oil in total to your bath water.

Compresses

Add 2-3 drops of each oil (7 drops max. in total) to 100ml (4fl oz) of hot water. Dip a clean piece of cotton in the liquid and apply it warm. When the compress cools, repeat using a new piece of cotton.

Inhalation

Add 2-3 drops of each oil (5 drops max. in total) to a bowl of hot water. Keep the bowl by your chair or bed.

Channel-opening techniques

You can enhance your acupressure treatment by "opening" the Channel you are about to treat – bringing it closer to the body surface. To do this, first look at the treatment plan to see which Channels to work on.

To open a Channel, you as "giver" need to ask the recipient to adopt the appropriate position, as shown below and on the following three pages. Some Channels are best opened by moving the arm (see below) and others respond best to moving the leg. Place your hands as illustrated, to provide a firm support in the position.

Opening the Channels in this way makes the points easier to work on and more sensitive to treatment. Many of these techniques also slightly stretch the tissues through which the Channels pass, which helps to unblock and smooth the flow of Qi. If the recipient is comfortable in the given position he/she can remain in it while you treat the acupoints. If not, just holding the position for two to three seconds before moving into a more comfortable one for treatment will help to open up the Channel and make your treatment more effective.

When you are working on more than one Channel in a treatment, you can either open the Channels first, then treat all the points, or open one Channel at a time, and work only on that Channel point before starting on the second, and so on. Do what is most convenient and most comfortable for both of you.

ARM POSITIONS

All the Channels on pages 32 and 33 are best opened with an arm movement, because they are most easily accessible in the arm. For the arm positions, keep your hand firmly but gently on the recipient's shoulder, to encourage him/her to let go of tension in the arms and relax into the treatment.

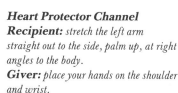

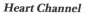

Heart Channel
Recipient: *stretch the left arm up and bend the elbow so the forearm is above the top of the head.*
Giver: *place your hands on the elbow and shoulder.*

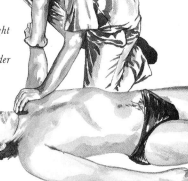

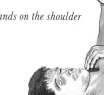

Heart Protector Channel
Recipient: *stretch the left arm straight out to the side, palm up, at right angles to the body.*
Giver: *place your hands on the shoulder and wrist.*

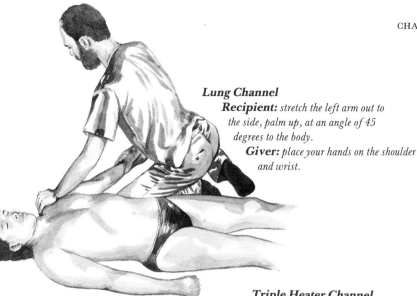

Lung Channel
Recipient: *stretch the left arm out to the side, palm up, at an angle of 45 degrees to the body.*

Giver: *place your hands on the shoulder and wrist.*

Triple Heater Channel
Recipient: *bend the left elbow at right angles, so the forearm lies across the belly.*

Giver: *place your hands on the shoulder and elbow.*

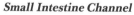

Large Intestine Channel
Recipient: *lie the left arm, palm down, beside the body.*

Giver: *place your hands on the shoulder and wrist.*

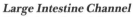

Small Intestine Channel
Recipient: *place the left arm across the chest, with the left hand on the right shoulder.*

Giver: *kneel on your right knee and place your hands on the shoulder and elbow.*

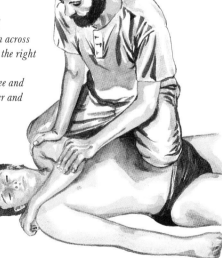

LEG POSITIONS

The Spleen, Liver, Kidney, Bladder, Gall Bladder, and Stomach Channels are all best opened by using a leg position.

If moving the leg also lifts the pelvis, hold your hand gently against the recipient's hip to keep the pelvis on the floor. Otherwise, just rest your hand on the belly for support.

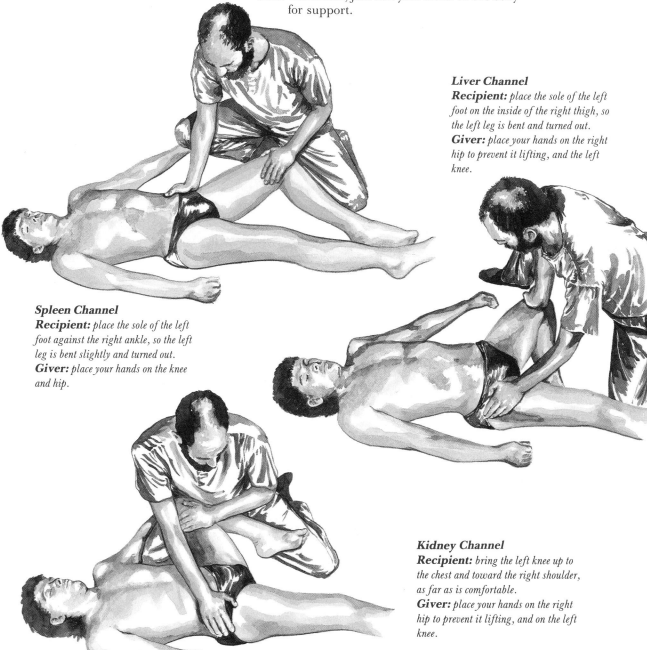

Liver Channel
Recipient: *place the sole of the left foot on the inside of the right thigh, so the left leg is bent and turned out.*
Giver: *place your hands on the right hip to prevent it lifting, and the left knee.*

Spleen Channel
Recipient: *place the sole of the left foot against the right ankle, so the left leg is bent slightly and turned out.*
Giver: *place your hands on the knee and hip.*

Kidney Channel
Recipient: *bring the left knee up to the chest and toward the right shoulder, as far as is comfortable.*
Giver: *place your hands on the right hip to prevent it lifting, and on the left knee.*

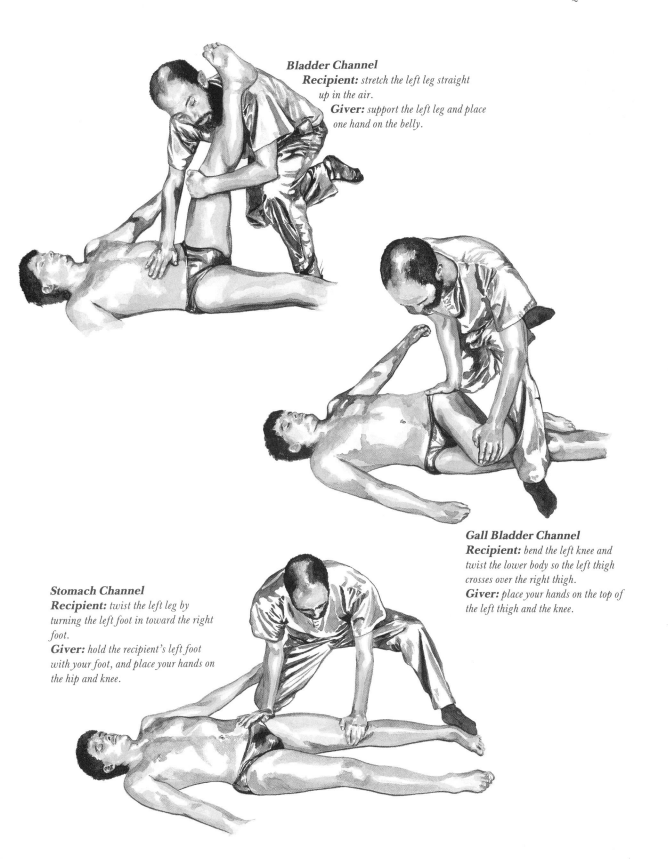

Bladder Channel
Recipient: *stretch the left leg straight up in the air.*
Giver: *support the left leg and place one hand on the belly.*

Gall Bladder Channel
Recipient: *bend the left knee and twist the lower body so the left thigh crosses over the right thigh.*
Giver: *place your hands on the top of the left thigh and the knee.*

Stomach Channel
Recipient: *twist the left leg by turning the left foot in toward the right foot.*
Giver: *hold the recipient's left foot with your foot, and place your hands on the hip and knee.*

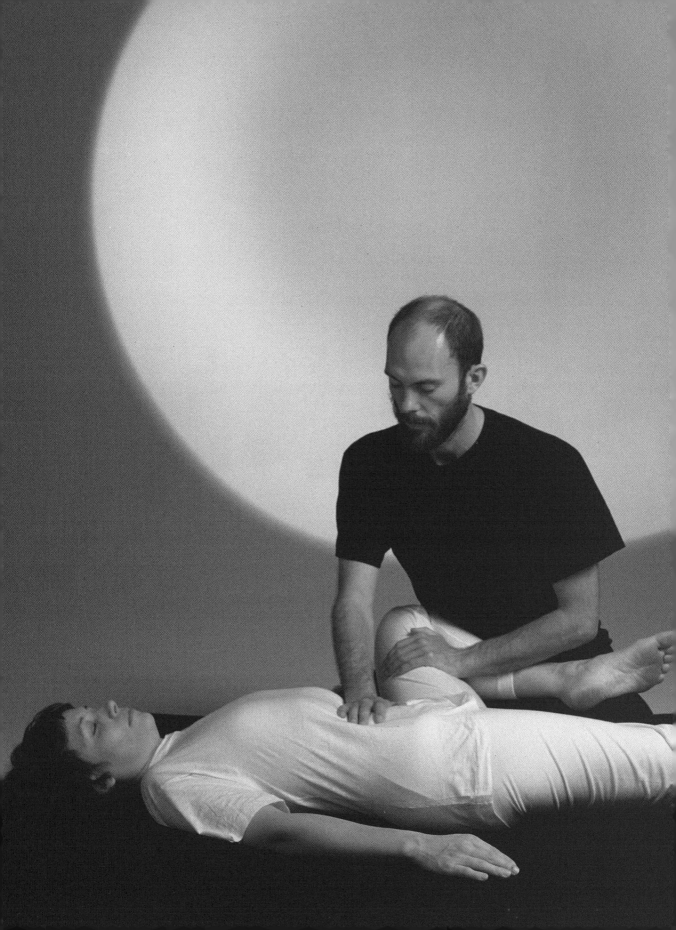

Part two

TREATING COMMON AILMENTS

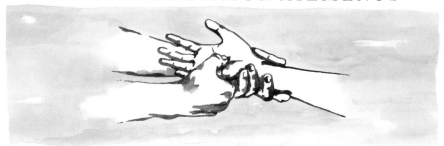

This section contains the treatment plans for common ailments, grouped according to where the symptoms occur. For example, the predominant symptoms of bronchitis are in the chest and respiratory system, so the treatment plan for bronchitis is under "Respiration". The introduction to each section explains both the Oriental and Western view of how each system functions and describes the internal and external factors such as diet and lifestyle that lead to disharmony.

The symptoms of each ailment are described in terms of Oriental and Western medicine. Each treatment plan describes the main points to treat, with an illustration and description of where to find them, and which pressure technique to use. Where additional points are recommended for treatments, they are shown on small diagrams at the foot of the page. Herbs and oils are recommended to complement each acupressure treatment, and details of how to use them are given on page 30. You should not treat some points during pregnancy, or if you have very high or very low blood pressure. Cautions are given for these whenever the pressure point is recommended in the treatment.

In *Major acupressure points* (pp. 24-27) the 12 points most commonly used in the treatments, are shown on detailed anatomical illustrations, The Channel networks are illustrated on pages 22-23. The *Summary of points* (pp. 88-90 helps you locate all the points used in the treatments). The illustrations on page 91 label the bones referred to in the instructions. The techniques of tonifying, calming, and dispersing the points are explained on page 29.

Ailments affecting general vitality come first, and then those affecting the two major systems of the body – the immune system and the nervous system. Then come ailments affecting the other systems: respiration; digestion; elimination; circulation, and finally reproduction. The treatments that follow are for ailments in the body's structure – the bones, joints, muscles, and sense organs (eyes and ears). These treatments are more local to the area of the symptoms. For example, for a pain in the ankle the treatment is to disperse St41, which is near the ankle joint, and moves Qi and Blood away from that area.

General vitality

Your inspiration, motivation, and zest for life are indicators of your life force. Our modern world makes many demands upon our energy and time and these draw on our inner reserves until eventually we run the risk of "burning out". This may start with fatigue and later can develop into dizziness, fainting, and collapse. According to Chinese medicine our vitality depends on the balance of Qi, Blood, and Mind, and these are influenced by our lifestyle. Both Western and Chinese medicine emphasize the need for adequate rest, exercise, social interaction, and a good diet. Acupressure helps improve your Blood and Qi circulation to counter life's pressures.

For how to use herbs and oils see page 30. For techniques for stimulating pressure points see page 29.

FATIGUE

The pattern of tiredness, general weakness, pale complexion, and weak voice represents Qi deficiency in Chinese medicine, and in Western medicine, mild depression. You need to stimulate the warming Yang Qi and nourishing Yin Qi. The most effective points are GV4 and CV4, and tonifying St36, Sp6, and LI4 may also be helpful.

CAUTION Never use Sp6 or LI4 during pregnancy.

Herbs *American ginseng*
Oils *Lavender*

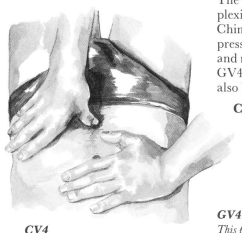

CV4

Locate this point 4 finger widths below the navel on the mid line of the belly. Tonify, or warm with an incense stick (see p. 29). This point is connected to the Liver, Spleen, and Kidney and invigorates the Yin Qi of the body.

GV4

This point is in the middle of the spine, between the 2nd and 3rd lumbar vertebrae. Tonify or warm it with an incense stick (see p. 29) to strengthen Kidney Yang Qi – the source of body warmth.

CAUTION Do not apply pressure in cases of sciatica or where there are disc problems.

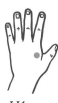

Note To give the recipient a greater feeling of comfort and balance, hold GV4 and CV4 simultaneously with your palms.

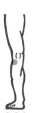

St36
(page 25)

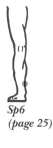

Sp6
(page 25)

LI4
(page 24)

FAINTING

The presence of numbness, weak tremors in the limbs, dizziness, and fainting represents blood deficiency in Chinese and Western medicine. On fainting, immediate first aid is required (see below), to revive the vital force. Then nourish and mobilize the blood circulation by treating GV26 and Sp6. It is also helpful to tonify CV4 and St36 and/or warm these points with an incense stick (see p. 29).

FIRST AID First loosen tight clothing and check there is a pulse and breathing is strong and regular. Raise the legs and if the person starts to vomit, roll on his/her side. Once awake, encourage the person to breathe slowly and deeply. Gradually raise into a sitting position and give sips of water. If unconsciousness lasts for two minutes or more, get the person to hospital.

Herbs 2-3 drops of cayenne pepper tincture (internally), smelling salts (check their pungency and hold strong-smelling salts at a distance)

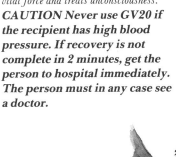

GV26

Find this point in the middle of the furrow between the nose and upper lip. Apply firm pressure with your thumbnail to tonify the point until the person comes round. Keep your other hand on GV20 on top of the head. This point revives the vital force and treats unconsciousness.

CAUTION Never use GV20 if the recipient has high blood pressure. If recovery is not complete in 2 minutes, get the person to hospital immediately. The person must in any case see a doctor.

Sp6

This is located 4 finger widths above the inside ankle bone, just behind the tibia. Tonify the point to strengthen the Spleen – the source of Blood and Qi.

CAUTION Never use this point during pregnancy.

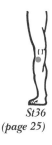

St36
(page 25)

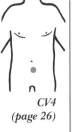

CV4
(page 26)

Nervous system

Our bodies' internal activities are delicately balanced, and depend on an intricate communication network of nerves to keep them working in harmony. According to both Chinese and Western medicine, disharmony in the nervous system can come from internal or external causes such as diet, stress, lack of activity, or hyperactivity. Acupressure and herbs help to calm or stimulate the system to keep it in balance.
For how to use herbs and oils see page 30. For techniques for stimulating pressure points see page 29.

HEADACHES

Headaches result from altered circulation in the head due to physical, emotional, or dietary causes. Imbalance in the Liver and Gall Bladder causes migraine headaches; Stomach and digestive imbalance causes forehead headaches. You need to disperse the stagnant Qi in the head and regulate Qi in the Organs. Treat points GB20, Yintang, Liv3, and St36.

CAUTION If the headache is severe or accompanied by dizziness or blurred vision, consult a doctor immediately.

Herbs *Peppermint*
Oils *Lavender, chamomile, marjoram*

CAUTION Never use marjoram oil during pregnancy.

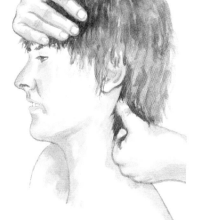

GB20
This is found at the base of the skull in the hairline, in a hollow between the front and back neck muscles, behind the bony prominence behind the ear. Disperse this point, directing your pressure toward the nose. This clears stagnant Qi in the head. Keep your other hand on the forehead to give support.

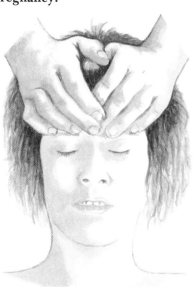

St36 and Liv3
Find St36 4 finger widths below the kneecap, outside the tibia. Tonify it to stimulate the digestive system, and relieve frontal headaches. Liv3 is in the furrow on the top of the foot between the 1st and 2nd toes, where the bones merge. Disperse this point to smooth the flow of Qi.

Yintang
This point is in the middle of the forehead, between the eyebrows. Disperse it with gentle fingertip pressure to shift stagnant Qi and to lift the cloudy mind that accompanies a headache.

STRESS AND TENSION

We think of stress as a negative force, but at normal levels it is essential for motivation. However, if we allow it to create tension it becomes harmful. In Chinese medicine tension is blocked Qi. You need to smooth the flow of Qi and transform tension from the upper body into vital Energy. Treat points Liv3, LI4, and GV20.

Herbs *Chamomile, clover blossom, motherwort*
Oils *Neroli, chamomile*

CAUTION Never use motherwort during pregnancy.

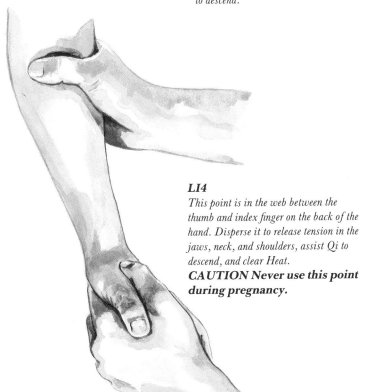

Liv3
Find this point in the furrow on the top of the foot between the 1st and 2nd toes, where the bones merge. Disperse it to smooth the flow of Qi, allowing stagnant Heat Energy in the upper body to descend.

LI4
This point is in the web between the thumb and index finger on the back of the hand. Disperse it to release tension in the jaws, neck, and shoulders, assist Qi to descend, and clear Heat.
CAUTION Never use this point during pregnancy.

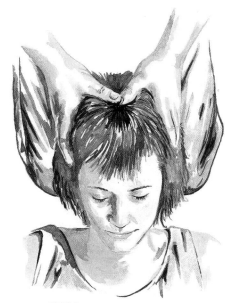

GV20
Locate this point in the middle of the top of the head, between the ears. Disperse it to clear tension in the head and cloudy thoughts, and raise pure, clear Qi. For immediate relief, place 1 drop of Bach Flower Rescue Remedy on this point.
CAUTION Never use this point if the recipient has high blood pressure.

ANXIETY AND WORRY

The familiar symptoms of anxiety range from nervous stomach to severe panic attacks. Western medicine sees it as a response to stress and treats it with sedatives and relaxation. Chinese medicine diagnoses an imbalance in the Spleen, Stomach, Heart, and Mind. You need to nourish the Spleen and Stomach, and calm the Mind. Treat points CV12, HP6, CV14, and H7. Tonification of St36 and Sp6 may also be helpful.

CAUTION For panic attacks seek professional guidance. Never use Sp6 during pregnancy.

Herbs *Chamomile, clover blossom, motherwort*
Oils *Bergamot, lavender, marjoram*

CAUTION Never use marjoram oil or motherwort during pregnancy.

CV12 and HP6

Find CV12 4 thumb widths above the navel on the mid line of the belly. Calm this point with your palm to stimulate the Spleen and Stomach to produce Qi and Blood, and induce calmness. HP6 is 2 thumb widths up from the palm side of the wrist, in the middle of the lower forearm. Calm this point to move congestion in the chest and Stomach and calm the Mind. Hold CV12 simultaneously.

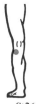
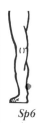

St36
(page 25)

Sp6
(page 25)

CV14 and H7

CV14 is 8 finger widths above the navel on the mid line of the belly. Calm this point with your palm to move Heart Qi and calm the Mind. Find H7 on the little finger side of the wrist crease. Calm this point to calm the Mind and improve Blood circulation in the Heart and chest.

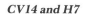

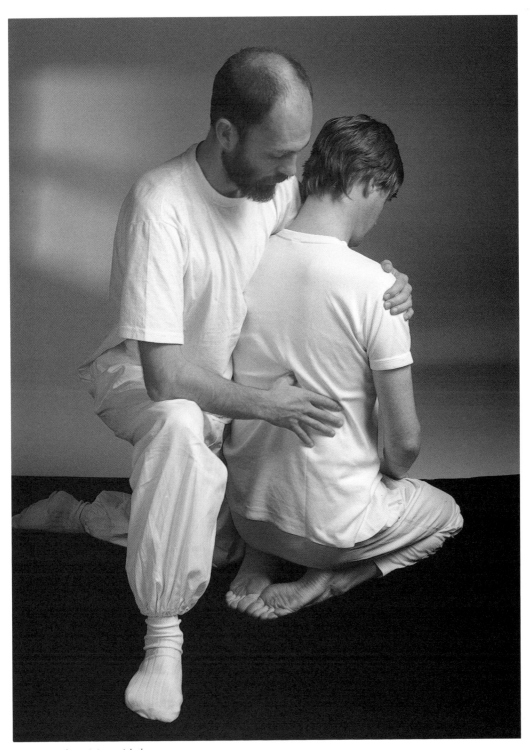

Supporting the recipient with the arm
during treatment brings added comfort.

DEPRESSION AND INSOMNIA

These do not always occur together, but the treatment is the same for both. Western medicine sees apathy, fatigue, poor appetite, palpitations, shortness of breath, and sleeplessness as depression, and prescribes antidepressants and sleeping pills. The Chinese interpretation is a deficiency of Heart Qi and Blood, due to lifestyle and emotional problems. Although insomnia and depression do not always occur together, the treatment for both is the same. Yin deficiency causes insomnia. You need to nourish the Blood and Qi, increase Yin, and calm the Mind. Treat points Sp6, B15, and CV14. Calming H7 and HP6 may also be helpful.

CAUTION For severe depression and/or insomnia, seek professional guidance.

Herbs *Passiflora, lavender, rosemary*
Oils *Sandalwood, chamomile, bergamot*

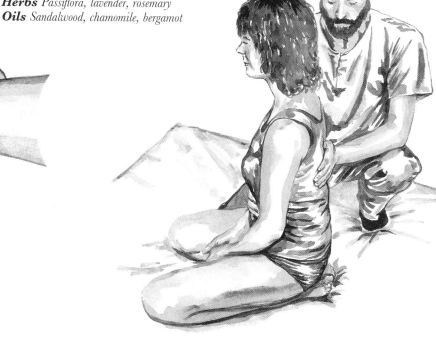

Sp6
This point is 4 finger widths above the inside ankle bone, just behind the tibia. Tonify it to stimulate production of Qi and Blood to nourish the Mind and Heart, and supplement Yin.
CAUTION Never use this point during pregnancy.

Bl5 and CV14
Locate B15 2 finger widths either side of the spine, level with the 5th and 6th thoracic vertebrae. Calm both points with your palm, and hold CV14 simultaneously. CV14 is 8 finger widths above the navel on the mid line of the belly. Calm this point with your palm. Both these treatments invigorate the circulation of Qi and Blood in the Heart, and calm the Mind.

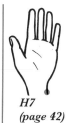

H7
(page 42)

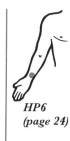

HP6
(page 24)

SHOCK

Shock is the body's reaction to traumatic incidents, either physical or emotional. In Chinese medicine it is the collapse of Yang Qi. The person will appear pale, cold, and clammy, with sweating, nausea and vomiting, anxiety, dizziness, and blurred vision, and possibly loss of consciousness. For mild cases of shock you need to tonify Yang Qi and nourish Yin Qi. Treat points K1 and CV6. Calming HP6 and tonifying St36 may also be helpful.

CAUTION In extreme cases shock can be fatal. Keep the sufferer warm and quiet. Call a doctor if concerned. Treat an unconscious person as an emergency – get him/her to hospital. Keep the legs raised and head turned to one side. Loosen clothing and cover with a blanket. Treat point GV26 (see p. 39).

Herbs *Cayenne pepper tincture, 2-3 drops; Bach Flower Remedy: Star of Bethlehem, 3 drops*
Oils *Melissa*

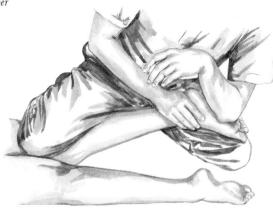

CV6

This point is 2 finger widths below the navel on the mid line of the belly. Tonify it gently with your thumb. This streng-thens Liver, Spleen, and Kidney Yin, and circulation, to overcome feelings of weakness.

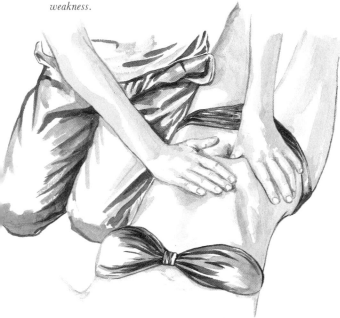

K1

Find this point in the crease in the middle of the ball of the foot, where the colour changes from the ball to the sole. Tonify it with your elbow to stimulate Kidney Yin and to revive consciousness.
CAUTION Never use this point if the recipient has low blood pressure.

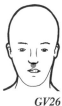

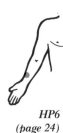

GV26
(page 39)

HP6
(page 24)

St36
(page 25)

Immune system

Atmospheric pollution, chemicals, poor diet, and stress all contribute to reducing our resistance to disease. This results in recurring infections, tiredness, insomnia, and apathy. Western medicine views this as a blend of psychosomatic symptoms and recurrent infection. Chinese medicine sees it as a weakness in protective Qi and nourishing Qi. Energy is trapped in the body surface, leaving it open to invasion by external energies such as Wind, Cold, Damp, and Heat. You need to strengthen the internal Organs and clear the trapped Energy from the body surface. *For how to use herbs and oils see page 30. For techniques for stimulating pressure points see page 29.*

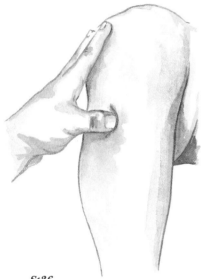

St36
This point is 4 finger widths below the kneecap, outside the tibia. Tonify it to strengthen Qi and Blood circulation to protect the body from infection.

STRENGTHENING THE SYSTEM
Use acupressure and herbs in conjunction with meditation, exercise, acupuncture, and a healthy diet to strengthen the immune system. Treat points B23, B20, B13, and St36. Tonifying LI4 may also be helpful.

CAUTION Seek professional help if there is weakness, weight loss, continual infection, and depression. Never use LI4 during pregnancy.

Herbs *Echinacea*
Chinese herbs *Huang Qi, Ling Zhi*

B23, B20, and B13
All these points are 2 finger widths either side of the spine. The B23 points are level with the 2nd and 3rd lumbar vertebrae. Tonify them to stimulate Kidney Qi – the source of Yin and Yang. Find B20 level with the 11th and 12th thoracic vertebrae and tonify to stimulate the Spleen – the source of Qi and Blood. The B13 points are level with the 3rd and 4th thoracic vertebrae. Tonify these to strengthen the Lungs.

● ● **B20**

● ● **B13**

LI4
(page 24)

POST VIRAL SYNDROME/ CHRONIC FATIGUE SYNDROME

Symptoms include feeling hot and then cold, headaches, lethargy, dizziness, and pain. In Western medicine the body is run-down, with a poor response to infection. Chinese medicine sees it as illness trapped half in and half out of the body. You need to disperse the trapped Qi to the body surface so it can be released. Treat points TH6, GV14, and GB41.

CAUTION A complete holistic programme is necessary for this condition. Seek professional guidance.

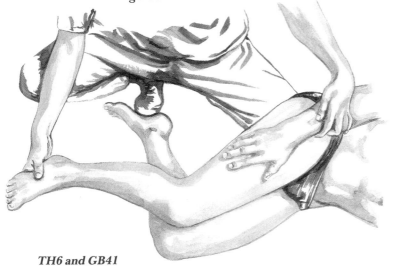

TH6 and GB41

TH6 is 4 finger widths above the wrist, on the back of the forearm. Disperse this point vigorously to remove stagnation and balance Qi in the upper, middle, and lower body. Find GB41 in the furrow between the 4th and 5th toes, just over the tendon on the top of the foot where the bones merge. Disperse it vigorously to clear Damp Heat, hold down rising Liver Qi, and clear the disease half in and half out of the body.

GV14

GV14 is on the back of the neck, between the 7th cervical and 1st thoracic vertebrae. Disperse this point vigorously to clear the Yang Channels and regulate temperature.

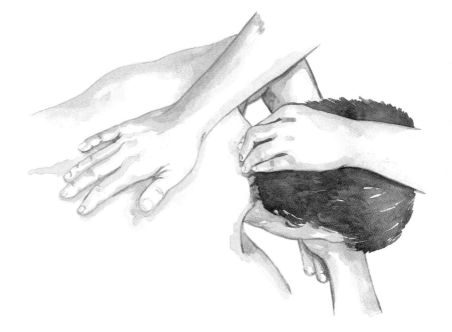

RECURRENT INFLUENZA

Western medicine regards this as re-infection due to a weakened immune system. It is sometimes treated with antibiotics. Chinese medicine sees it as weak Lung Qi and weak protective Qi at the body surface, due to poor diet, inappropriate lifestyle, and stress. You need to strengthen the Lungs and protective Qi and clear the Qi trapped in the body surface. Treat points TH5 and Lu7. Tonifying B13, LI4, and CV6 may also be helpful.

CAUTION A complete holistic programme is necessary for this condition. Seek professional guidance. Never use LI4 during pregnancy.

Herbs *Marshmallow root, mullein*
Oils *Lavender, pine*

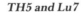

TH5 and Lu7

TH5 is 2 thumb widths above the wrist, on the back of the forearm. Disperse this point to clear the body surface and protect it from invasion by external energies such as Wind. Find Lu7 2 finger widths above the wrist crease on the thumb side, just off the radius bone. Disperse it to clear the body surface, strengthen the Lungs, and stimulate protective Qi.

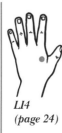

*B13
(page 46)*

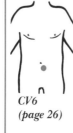

*LI4
(page 24)*

*CV6
(page 26)*

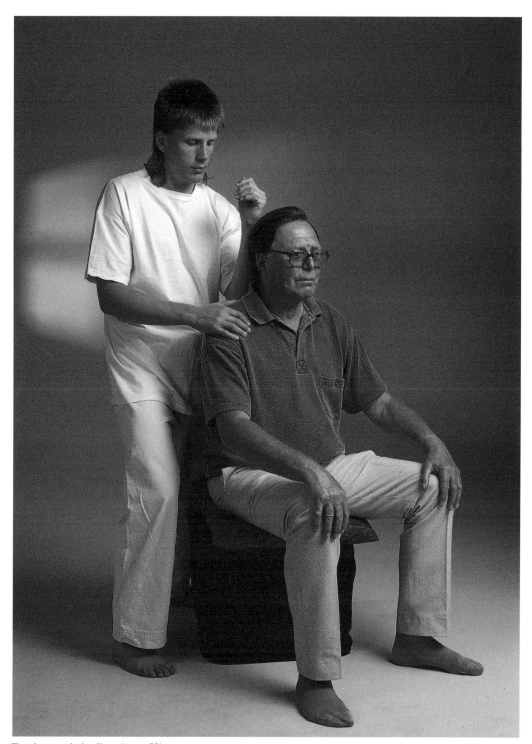

Tonifying with the elbow (see p. 29).

Respiration

The polluted air we breathe and the congesting foods we eat (junk foods, dairy products, and so on) cause and aggravate respiratory diseases. In the view of Western medicine they result from infection, allergic responses, and/or intrinsic weakness. According to Chinese medicine they are caused by external factors such as Wind, Cold, and Damp, which invade when there is internal weakness caused by poor diet. It is vital to strengthen the Lungs and clear the body surface and the invading element.

For how to use herbs and oils see page 30. For techniques for stimulating pressure points see page 29.

COLDS

Western medicine views a cold as a generalized upper airways infection. In Chinese medicine it signifies invasion by Wind and Cold, causing fever, headache, stiff neck, aversion to wind and cold, vague joint pains, but no sweating. You need to disperse the Wind and Cold and strengthen the Lungs. Treat points Lu7 and GV14. Dispersing LI4 and GB20 may also be helpful.

CAUTION Never use LI4 during pregnancy.

Herbs *Ginger and cinnamon twig tea*
Oils *Black pepper, eucalyptus*

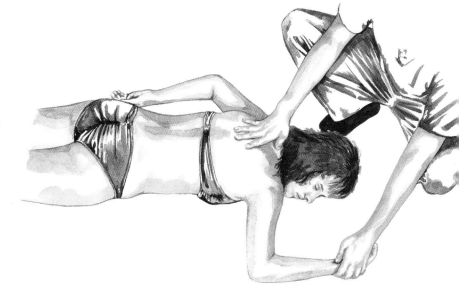

Lu7and GV14

Find Lu7 2 finger widths above the wrist crease, on the thumb side of the radius bone. Disperse this point to clear the body surface and strengthen the Lungs. GV14 is on the back of the neck between the 7th cervical and 1st thoracic vertebrae. Disperse it to clear the Yang Channels and eliminate Wind and Cold.

L14
(page 24)

GB20
(page 27)

INFLUENZA

Each year brings with it another influenza virus, responsible for flu outbreaks, according to Western medicine. The Chinese view of flu is an invasion of Wind and Heat in the body surface and Lungs. This results in fever, thirst, headaches, sweating, and stuffiness in the chest and nasal passages. You need to disperse the Wind and Heat and strengthen the Lungs. Treat points LI11 and Lu10. Dispersing LI4 and GB20 may also be helpful.

CAUTION Never use LI4 during pregnancy.

Herbs Peppermint, elderower, dandelion and burdock
Oils Lavender, lemon

CAUTION Only use lemon oil in very low dilutions. Do not use if you have a sensitive skin.

LI11

This point is at the end of the outside elbow crease, and is most easily found with the elbow bent. Disperse it to clear Wind and Heat from the body surface.

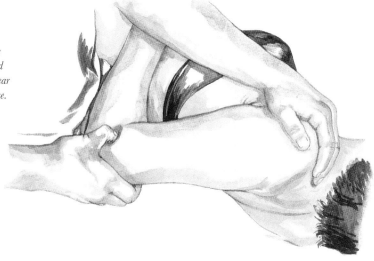

Lu10

Find this point 2 finger widths down from the wrist crease, along the palm side of the thumb. Disperse it to clear Heat from the Lungs.

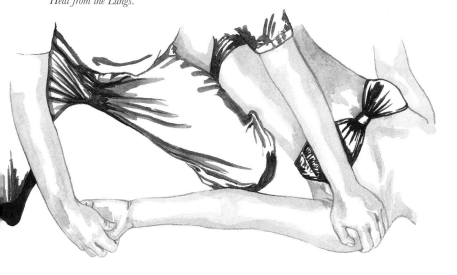

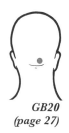

L14
(page 24)

GB20
(page 27)

SINUSITIS

Allergy and infection are responsible for inflammation of the sinus, according to Western medicine. In Chinese medicine it is the invasion and stagnation of Wind, Cold, and Damp, and Lung weakness that is responsible, resulting in a runny nose, feeling of stuffiness, and excess phlegm. You need to open the nasal passages, clear the body surface, and strengthen the Lungs. Treat LI20 and Bitong. Dispersing Yintang, LI4, and GB20 may also be helpful.

CAUTION Never use LI4 during pregnancy.

Herbs *Marshmallow*
Oils *Pine, lavender, basil*

CAUTION Never use basil oil during pregnancy.

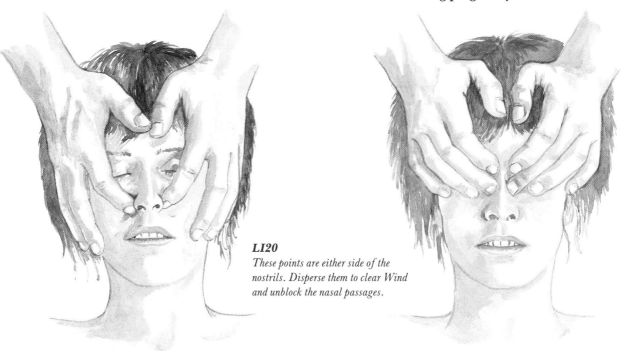

LI20
These points are either side of the nostrils. Disperse them to clear Wind and unblock the nasal passages.

Bitong
These points are halfway down either side of the bridge of the nose. Disperse them to clear Wind and Cold and clear the nasal passages.

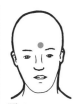

Yintang
(page 40)

LI4
(page 53)

GB20
(page 27)

SORE THROAT

In Western medicine a sore throat often accompanies colds or flu. On its own it is a symptom of being run-down. In Chinese medicine it represents Heat in the Lungs and upper airways. You need to cool the Lungs and clear Heat from the body. Treat points Lu11 and LI4.

Herb*s Sage, honey and lemon juice tea*

CAUTION Never use sage oil in pregnancy.

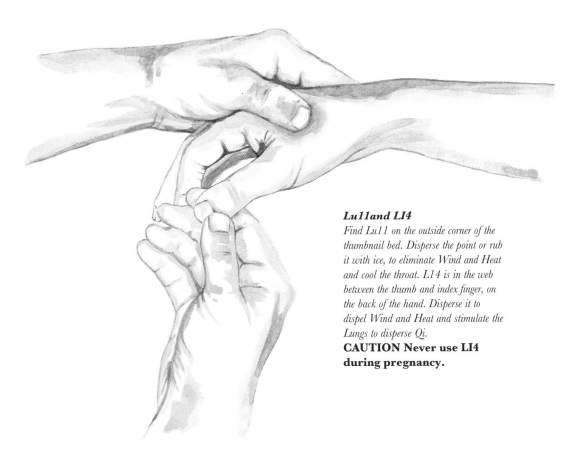

Lu11and LI4
Find Lu11 on the outside corner of the thumbnail bed. Disperse the point or rub it with ice, to eliminate Wind and Heat and cool the throat. L14 is in the web between the thumb and index finger, on the back of the hand. Disperse it to dispel Wind and Heat and stimulate the Lungs to disperse Qi.
CAUTION Never use LI4 during pregnancy.

ASTHMA

An asthma attack is an acute (short-term) condition. A person who suffers recurrent attacks has chronic asthma. According to Western medicine it is due to a hypersensitivity of the bronchial tubes, which constrict causing difficulty in breathing, wheezing, and distress, after which there is often a productive cough. In Chinese medicine asthma signifies weakness of the Lungs and Kidneys, coupled with bouts of acute invasion of Wind and Cold. You need to relax the chest, clear the Lungs, and strengthen the Kidneys, which pull Energy down into the body. Treat Lu6 and Ding Chuan. After an attack, tonify B13 and B23, and disperse LI4.

Natural medicine has a great deal to offer asthma. Seek guidance from a professional practitioner.

CAUTION For acute breathlessness see a doctor immediately. Never use LI4 during pregnancy.

Herbs *Elecampane root, nettles, thyme*
Oils *Lavender, pine, ginger*

Lu6

This point is 7 thumb widths above the wrist crease on the inside of the forearm, in line with the thumb. Disperse this point to regulate the Lungs, and make Lung Qi descend to stop the attack.

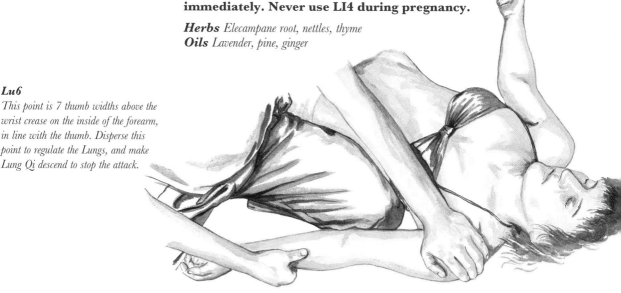

Ding Chuan

Find these points half a thumb width either side of GV14, between the 7th cervical and 1st thoracic vertebrae. Disperse the points and then apply ginger oil. This stops the attack and releases tightness in the chest.

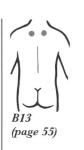

B13
(page 55)

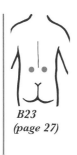

B23
(page 27)

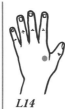
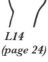

L14
(page 24)

BRONCHITIS

Western medicine regards this as an inflammation of the mucous membranes of the bronchial tubes, with short, rapid, wheezy breathing, a productive cough, and infection. In Chinese medicine it results from an imbalance in the water metabolism and weakness in the Lungs. You need to strengthen the Lungs, open the chest, and regulate the water metabolism. Treat points CV17, B13, and Lu1 for acute or chronic cases, and Lu9 for chronic cases. Tonifying Sp6 and St36 may also be helpful.

CAUTION Use acupressure as a back-up to professional guidance. Never use Sp6 during pregnancy.

Herbs *Wild cherry bark, elecampane root, echinacea, mullein, lungwort, saw palmetto*
Oils *Lavender, pine*

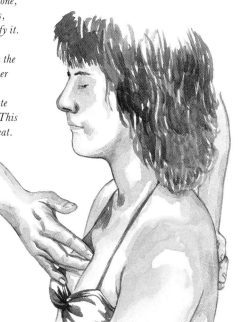

CV17 and B13

CV17 is in the middle of the breastbone, between the nipples. In acute attacks, calm the point. In chronic cases tonify it. This point stimulates Lung Qi and moves the mucus. Find B13 between the shoulder blades, 2 finger widths either side of the 3rd and 4th thoracic vertebrae. Disperse this point in acute attacks and tonify in chronic cases. This strengthens the Lungs and clears Heat.

Lu1 and Lu9

Lu1 is below the bony prominence in front of the shoulder, under the shoulder end of the collar bone. Disperse in acute attacks and tonify in chronic cases. This point disperses fullness in the chest and moves mucus. Find Lu9 in the wrist crease at the base of the thumb, on the palm side. Tonify it to strengthen Lung Yin and clear Phlegm.

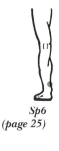

Sp6
(page 25)

St36
(page 25)

Shiatsu techniques to improve respiration

The tensions of our modern lifestyle, and poor posture aggravated by long periods of sitting, all contribute to bad breathing habits. Most of us breathe with only a small part of our lungs. If you have an inherent lung weakness, the inability to breathe slowly and deeply into the lower regions of the lungs may make you more prone to respiratory ailments. The following shiatsu techniques are excellent for improving breathing.

Rib pressing
The recipient should lie face up. You will probably find it most comfortable to kneel on one knee beside him/her. Spread your hands over the lower ribs, ensuring that your hands cover a broad expanse of rib cage. As the recipient breathes in, let your hands accommodate the expansion of the rib cage, while maintaining contact. On the outward breath apply light pressure to encourage a fuller exhalation. Repeat this three or four times, allowing the recipient to dictate the breathing rhythm.

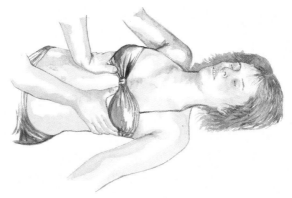

ACUPRESSURE TECHNIQUES TO IMPROVE RESPIRATION

According to Chinese medicine, breathing depends on the Kidneys as well as the Lungs, as the Kidney "pulls down" Lung Qi. Treating CV6 and CV17 simultaneously stimulates this Kidney function. Concentrate on the connection between the two points (see p. 28), to increase the depth of breathing.

CV6 and CV17
Find CV6 2 finger widths below the navel, on the mid line of the belly. Tonify it to clear Damp in the Lung, and strengthen the Kidney and the rest of the body. CV17 is on the breastbone, midway between the nipples. Calm this point to stimulate Lung Qi and clear mucus.

Digestion

In our fast-food society we do not allow ourselves enough time to eat and digest our food. Our digestive systems rebel against the onslaught of convenience foods, resulting in sluggish digestion and stagnation in the bowel. Symptoms range from poor appetite to ulcers and even cancer. Western doctors are now recognizing the need for sensible eating habits. In Chinese medicine eating regular balanced meals and allowing time to digest them is essential to health. Stimulation of the Spleen and Stomach, which transform food and liquid into Qi and Blood, improves digestion.

CAUTION All these conditions may be acute (short-term) or chronic (long-term). If symptoms are severe, seek professional guidance.

For how to use herbs and oils see page 30. For techniques for stimulating pressure points see page 29.

WEAK DIGESTION/LOSS OF APPETITE

If you tend to get indigestion after eating, however carefully you choose and eat your food, you may have weak digestion. Symptoms may include general weakness, loss of appetite, abdominal bloating, wind, and loose stools. The Western interpretation is mild depression. In Chinese medicine it is weakness in the Spleen and Stomach. You need to strengthen and warm the Spleen and Stomach. Treat points B23 and B20. Tonifying GV4, Sp6, St36, and St25 may also be helpful.

CAUTION Never use Sp6 during pregnancy.

Herbs *Fennel, meadowsweet, wood betony, cardamom, cinnamon*
Oils *Chamomile, bergamot*

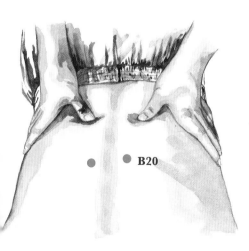

● ● **B20**

B23 and B20
All these points are 2 finger widths either side of the spine. B23 is level with the 2nd and 3rd lumbar vertebrae. Tonify these points to increase Kidney Yang - the source of body warmth. The B20 points are level with the 11th and 12th thoracic vertebrae. Tonify them to strengthen the Spleen, helping digestion and the formation of Qi and Blood.

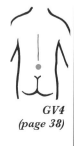

GV4
(page 38)

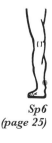

Sp6
(page 25)

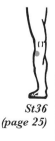

St36
(page 25)

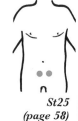

St25
(page 58)

INDIGESTION AND NAUSEA

Rapid eating and overconsumption leads to distension, fullness, belching, bloating, pain in the abdomen, and vomiting. In Chinese and Western medicine the cause is food stagnation due to overeating or rapid eating without chewing properly. You need to disperse the stagnation and stimulate the Spleen, Stomach, and the circulation in the bowel. Treat points CV12, Liv13, and St25. Calming HP6 and dispersing St36 may also be helpful.

CAUTION Do not ask the sufferer to lie on his/her back if vomiting is still likely.

Herbs *Peppermint, ginger, caraway, alfalfa*
Oils *Lavender*

CV12 and Liv13
Find CV12 4 thumb widths above the navel on the mid line of the belly. Disperse this point to stimulate the Spleen and Stomach, move stagnation, and stop vomiting. Liv13 is below the 11th rib, at the side and bottom of the rib cage, in line with the hip bone. Disperse this point to move stagnation in the Stomach and stimulate the Spleen.

St25
Locate these points 2 thumb widths either side of the navel. Disperse them to stimulate the circulation in the bowel.

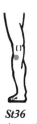

*St36
(page 59)*

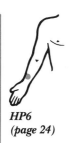

*HP6
(page 24)*

STOMACH ACIDITY

Poor diet, overeating, and stress can all lead to excessive acid in the Stomach, causing intense pain, regurgitation, heartburn, and nausea. Western doctors prescribe antacids, which encourage the Stomach to produce more acid, making it more acidic in the long term. Avoid them if possible: it is better to adjust your diet. The Chinese interpretation is stagnation and excessive Stomach Heat. You need to remove stagnation, clear Heat, and cool and regulate the Stomach. Treat points St43, St44, St41, and St36.

Herbs *Dill, chamomile*
Oils *Bergamot, chamomile*

St43 and St44

St43 is in the furrow between the 2nd and 3rd toes, where the bones merge on top of the foot. Disperse this point to cool the Stomach. Find St44 in the web at the base of the 2nd and 3rd toes, on top of the foot. Disperse it to remove fullness and Heat from the Stomach.

St41 and St36

Locate St41 in the middle of the ankle joint, on the front of the ankle. Disperse this point to clear Heat from the Stomach. St36 is 4 finger widths below the kneecap, outside the tibia. Disperse it to regulate the Stomach and invigorate circulation.

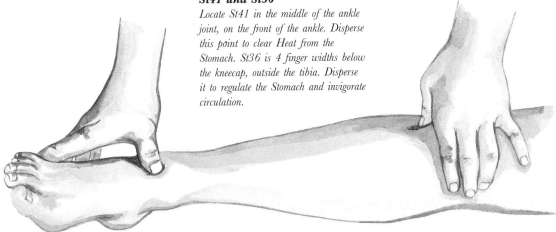

FLATULENCE AND BLOATING

This is an accumulation of gas in the stomach and/or bowel that is expelled via the mouth or anus. There is often abdominal pain, restlessness, and irritability. According to Western medicine the cause is food fermenting in the digestive tract. The Chinese interpretation is stagnation of Damp Heat and a Liver-Spleen disharmony that causes wind. You need to regulate the Liver and Spleen and clear Damp Heat. Treat points Sp4, Liv3, and St36. Dispersing CV12 and calming HP6 may also be helpful.

Herbs *In cooking marjoram, coriander, fennel, aniseed, cardamom, dill, cumin. As tea: peppermint, catnip, lemon balm*
Oils *Chamomile, fennel, bergamot, cardamom*

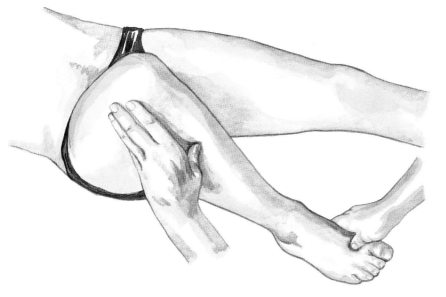

Liv3 and St36

Find Liv3 in the furrow between the 1st and 2nd toes, where the bones merge on top of the foot. Disperse this point to soothe the Liver and regulate Qi circulation. St36 is 4 finger widths below the kneecap, outside the tibia. Disperse it to regulate the Stomach and Spleen, eliminate wind and Damp, and stimulate circulation.

Sp4

This point is on the inside arch of the foot, just under the base of the big toe. Disperse it to regulate the middle of the body and calm the Stomach and Damp Heat.

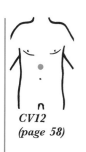

**CV12
(page 58)**

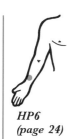

**HP6
(page 24)**

Elimination

The bowel and bladder remove waste matter and absorb any essential nutrients remaining. The kidney filters liquids to maintain fluid levels in the body. In Western medicine elimination problems are related to diet, infection, and irritable bowel or bladder. Chinese medicine recognizes the interplay between the liquid content of the bladder and bowel and that of the food eaten.

For how to use herbs and oils see page 30. For techniques for stimulating pressure points see page 29.

CONSTIPATION

The bowels do not open regularly or completely and stools are dry and hard. According to Western medicine this may be due to excessive water absorption, spasm or lack of tone in the muscles of the bowel wall, a low-fibre diet, bowel obstruction, or habitual neglect of the desire to "go". The Chinese view of a short-term problem may be excessive internal Heat from hot spicy food or emotional problems. A long-term problem is more likely to arise from weak Qi and Blood. You need to balance the Colon function. Treat B25 and B18: tonify for a long-term condition and disperse if the problem is short term. Treating TH6 and St25 may also be helpful.

Herbs *Basil, dandelion root, black sesame seeds*
Oils *Rosemary*

CAUTION Avoid purgative medicines. If your regular bowel movement patterns change or if constipation occurs suddenly, consult your doctor.

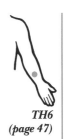

B25 and B18
These points are all 2 finger widths either side of the spine. The B25 points, level with the 4th and 5th lumbar vertebrae, balance the Colon function. Disperse them to remove Heat, and tonify to strengthen weak Qi and Blood. Find B18 level with the 9th and 10th thoracic vertebrae. Tonify them to regulate the Liver and circulation. Disperse to disperse stagnant Qi and stagnation in the Colon.

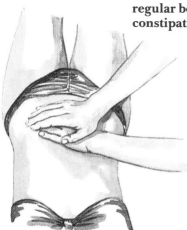

Wave rocking
Kneel and place one hand on top of the other on the right side of the belly, then produce a wave-like rocking motion with your hands, working from the heels of your palms to your fingertips. The rhythm should be slow and graceful. It assists the movement of the bowel contents.

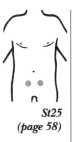

TH6
(page 47)   *St25*
                     (page 58)

DIARRHOEA

Western medicine diagnoses looseness of the bowels as malabsorption or excess fluid and mucus from the bowel lining due to diet, nervousness, or infection, and treats it with antibiotics or kaolin and morphine, for example. According to Chinese medicine it is lack of warming Yang Qi in the Spleen, Stomach, and Kidney, or excessive intake of Damp foods. Treat points B23, B22, B20, and St37, tonifying for a long-standing condition, and dispersing if onset is recent. Treatment of B25, CV4, St36, Sp9, and St25 may also be helpful.

CAUTION Severe cases may result in dehydration. If diarrhoea persists for more than 24 hours (3-4 hours in children), consult your doctor.

Herbs *Cinnamon, hawthorn berries, prickly ash bark, raspberry leaves, nettles, huckleberry, rosehips*
Oils *Lavender, chamomile, cypress*

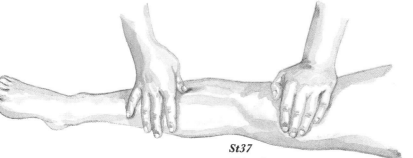

B23, B22, and B20
These points are all 2 finger widths either side of the spine. The B23 points are level with the 2nd and 3rd lumbar vertebrae. They strengthen the Kidney – the source of Yang Qi – and eliminate Damp. Find B22 level with the 1st and 2nd lumbar vertebrae. They regulate the movement of water in the lower body. The B20 points are level with the 11th and 12th thoracic vertebrae, and regulate the Spleen and eliminate Damp.

St37
This point is 8 finger widths below the kneecap, outside the tibia, and removes Damp Heat from the bowel.

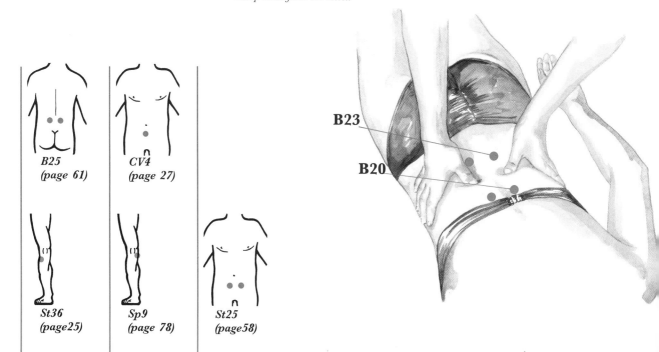

B23

B20

B25
(page 61)

CV4
(page 27)

St36
(page 25)

Sp9
(page 78)

St25
(page 58)

CYSTITIS

Pain in the lower pelvis and back, frequent, painful urination, bad-smelling, cloudy urine, and possibly fever, indicate cystitis. The Western view is inflammation of the bladder due to infection, and treatments include medication, rest, and drinking plenty of water. Chinese doctors see it as an accumulation of Damp Heat in the Bladder due to poor diet, emotional upset, or weakness of Qi and Blood. You need to clear the Damp Heat and promote urination. Treat points St29, CV3, and B32. Dispersing B54 and B60 may also help.

CAUTION Never use B60 during pregnancy.

Herbs *Cleavers, marshmallow, dandelion root, nettles, couchgrass, corn silk, ginger root, saw palmetto berries*

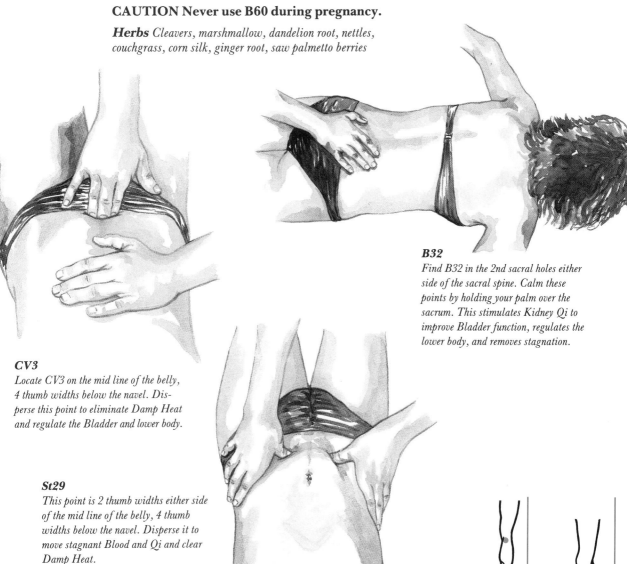

B32
Find B32 in the 2nd sacral holes either side of the sacral spine. Calm these points by holding your palm over the sacrum. This stimulates Kidney Qi to improve Bladder function, regulates the lower body, and removes stagnation.

CV3
Locate CV3 on the mid line of the belly, 4 thumb widths below the navel. Disperse this point to eliminate Damp Heat and regulate the Bladder and lower body.

St29
This point is 2 thumb widths either side of the mid line of the belly, 4 thumb widths below the navel. Disperse it to move stagnant Blood and Qi and clear Damp Heat.

B54
(page 85)

B60
(page 83)

Circulation

Our bodies contain an enormous amount of fluid: nearly 5 litres (8 pints) of blood and 10 litres (16 pints) of lymph, which must circulate continuously to nourish the body and carry away waste products. Western doctors see poor circulation as a result of smoking, bad diet, high cholesterol, lack of exercise, or congenital weakness in the blood vessels. Treatment ranges from change of diet to medication and surgery. The Chinese also acknowledge the impact of lifestyle on circulation, but emphasize as well the relationship between Qi and Blood. Qi moves the Blood and the Blood nourishes Qi. You need to strengthen and move Qi and nourish and invigorate the Blood.

For how to use herbs and oils see page 30. For techniques for stimulating pressure points see page 29.

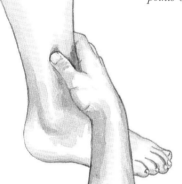

GB39
This is a special point for bone marrow, 4 finger widths above the outside ankle bone, in front of the fibula. Tonify it to invigorate the Yang Channels of the legs.

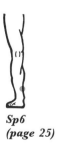

Sp6
(page 25)

COLD HANDS AND FEET

Cold extremities may be a seasonal or regular occurrence. The Western explanation is spasm in the smaller arteries in the limbs, possibly due to nervous influences that are aggravated by cold weather restricting circulation. The Chinese see it as a weakness of Blood, Yang Qi, and circulation. You need to tonify Qi and Blood and promote circulation. Treat points GB39 and LI10. Tonifying LI4, HP6, St36, Sp6, and Liv3 may also be helpful.

CAUTION Never use LI4 or Sp6 during pregnancy.

Herbs *Dried ginger, cinnamon, garlic*
Oils *Black pepper*

LI10
Find Li10 2 thumb widths below the crease on the outside of the elbow, in line with the middle of the back of the wrist. This point governs the Yang Channels of the arms. Tonify it to invigorate circulation.

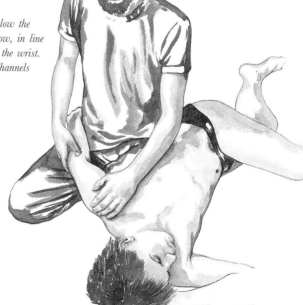

LI4
(page 24)

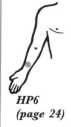

HP6
(page 24)

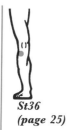

St36
(page 25)

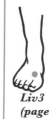

Liv3
(page 25)

HAEMORRHOIDS

Haemorrhoids, or piles, are the veins in the lower bowel that become distended and inflamed and may bleed. The Western view is that they result from a sedentary lifestyle, overeating and constipation, or pregnancy. They may also be a symptom of disease higher up in the digestive tract. The treatment involves diet, exercise, medication, and possibly surgery. According to Chinese medicine they are due to poor lifestyle and diet, which cause Damp Heat in the bowel, Blood stagnation in the pelvis, and sinking Qi. You need to invigorate Qi and Blood circulation and raise Qi. Treat points GV20, GV1, and B57.

CAUTION If the piles are bleeding, see your doctor.

Herbs *Powdered yarrow, bayberry, pilewort, or comfrey root, as a poultice, or mixed with oil, and applied to the piles. Yellow dock and nettles for bleeding piles, applied similarly.*
Oils *Cypress, marigold, myrrh*

CAUTION Never use marigold or myrrh oils or bayberry during pregnancy.

GV1
This point is on the mid line, halfway between the coccyx and anus. Calm it by placing your palm over the area. This removes blockage and stagnation in the Conception and Governing Channels, and reduces pain.

B57
Locate this point in the middle of the back of the calf, at the junction of the muscle and tendon. Tonify it to move Blood stagnation in the pelvis.

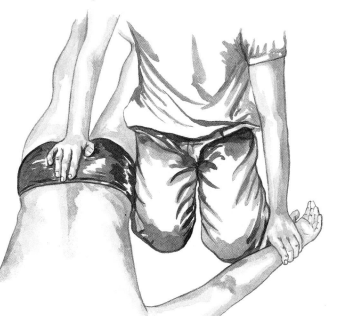

GV20
Find this point in the middle of the top of the head, between the ears. Tonify it to raise Qi.
CAUTION *Never use this point if the recipient has high blood pressure.*

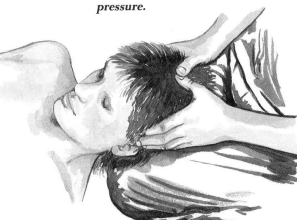

Reproductive system

The reproductive system is delicately regulated by the hormonal system and blood circulation. These internal rhythms are affected by physical, emotional, and nutritional factors.

For how to use herbs and oils see page 30. For techniques for stimulating pressure points see page 29.

MENSTRUAL PAIN

Painful menstruation is very common, and Western medicine diagnoses a range of causes, including anaemia, inflammation, imperfect development of the uterus and ovaries, fibroids, endometriosis, and cancer. In Chinese medicine exposure to cold, excess cold food, and weakness of Qi and Blood can disturb menstruation. You need to regulate Qi and Blood and the internal organs, especially the Liver, Spleen, and Kidneys.

CAUTION If menstrual pain is severe you should seek professional guidance.

PAIN BEFORE THE PERIOD

Bloating, swollen breasts, irritability, and depression often accompany the pain. In Chinese medicine this suggests stagnation of Liver Qi. Treat points Sp8, Liv3, and CV6. Calming CV3 may also be helpful.

Herbs *Wild yam, caraway, ginger root*
Oils *Cypress, melissa*

Sp8
Find Sp8 4 finger widths below the inside of the knee joint, between the calf muscle and the tibia. Disperse this point to circulate the Blood and remove stagnation in the uterus.

Liv3
This point is in the furrow on top of the foot between the 1st and 2nd toes, where the bones merge. Disperse it to regulate the circulation of Qi and Blood.

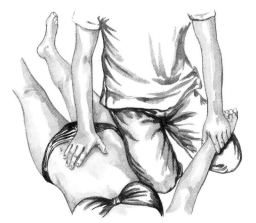

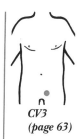

CV6
Find CV6 2 finger widths below the navel on the mid line of the belly. Calm this point by placing your palm over it, to regulate Qi circulation and help clear the pain.

CV3
(page 63)

PAIN DURING THE PERIOD

The pain is often severe, radiating to the lower back and thighs, and worse if you press the lower abdomen. Clots and heavy flow often accompany the pain. In Chinese medicine this is stagnation of Blood due to a Spleen-Liver disharmony. Treat points Sp6 and St36. Calming CV6 and CV4, and tonifying B23, may also be helpful.

Herbs *As for before the period, and motherwort*
Oils *As for before the period*

St36
Find this point 4 finger widths below the kneecap, outside the tibia. Disperse it to circulate Qi and Blood.

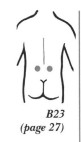

Sp6
This point is 4 finger widths above the inside ankle bone, just behind the tibia. Disperse it to regulate the Yin Channels in the legs, and Qi and Blood in the uterus.

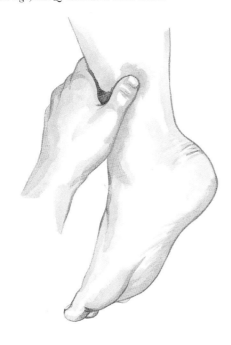

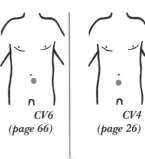

CV6
(page 66)

CV4
(page 26)

B23
(page 27)

PAIN AFTER THE PERIOD

The pain is often better with warmth and pressure. Scanty flow, palpitations, dizziness, and weakness often accompany the pain. In Chinese medicine this signifies Qi and Blood weakness. Treat points B23, B20, and B18. Tonifying Sp6, CV4, and St36 may also be helpful.

Herbs and oils *As for before the period*

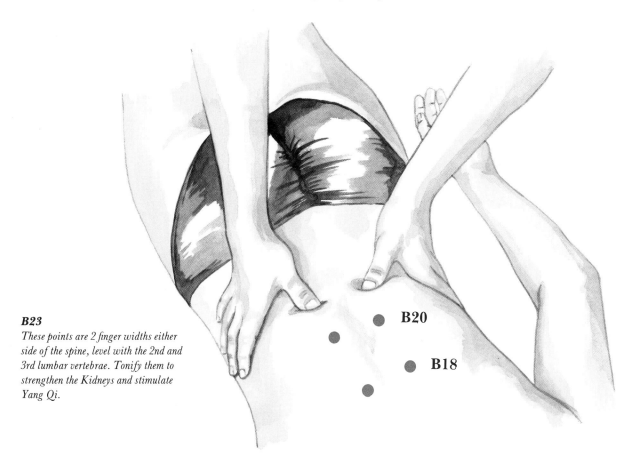

B23
These points are 2 finger widths either side of the spine, level with the 2nd and 3rd lumbar vertebrae. Tonify them to strengthen the Kidneys and stimulate Yang Qi.

B20
Find these points 2 finger widths either side of the spine, level with the 11th and 12th thoracic vertebrae. Tonify them to strengthen the Spleen – the source of Qi and Blood.

B18
The B18 points are 2 finger widths either side of the spine, level with the 9th and 10th thoracic vertebrae. Tonify them to disperse stagnant Qi, and regulate the Liver and circulation.

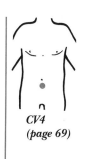

CV4
(page 69)

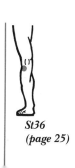

St36
(page 25)

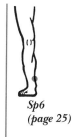

Sp6
(page 25)

HEAVY MENSTRUATION

If the blood is deep red and smells, and is accompanied by feelings of restlessness, Chinese medicine sees it as Liver Qi stagnation, creating Heat and excess flow of Blood. This is often a result of emotional stress.

If the blood is light-coloured and is accompanied by tiredness, the Spleen is not controlling the Blood in the vessels, due to worry or poor diet.

For both conditions treat points Sp1 and CV4. Disperse Liv3 to regulate the Liver and improve its ability to store Blood, and smooth the flow of Qi. Tonifying Liv1, on the inside corner of the nail bed of the big toe, may also be helpful.

Herbs *Raspberry leaf, squaw vine, agrimony, madder root, tincture of fresh shepherd's purse*
Oils *Geranium, cypress*

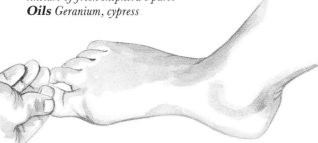

Sp1

This point is on the outside corner of the nail bed of the big toe. Tonify it strongly using your thumbnail (see p. 29), or warm it with an incense stick. This calms the Spleen and Stomach and improves the Spleen's ability to control the Blood.

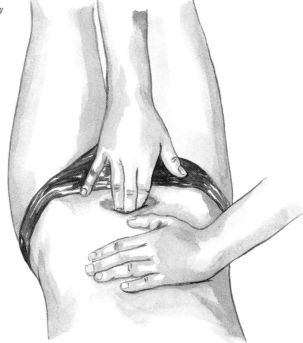

CV4

This point also reaches the Liver, Spleen, Kidney, and Conception Channels. Find it 4 finger widths below the navel on the mid line of the belly and tonify it to check the flow of Blood.

Liv3
(page 60)

Liv1
(page 90)

PRE-MENSTRUAL SYNDROME

This can include irritability, depression, breast distension, a craving for sweets, lower abdominal bloating, and nausea. In Western medicine this is due to hormonal imbalance and psychological factors. In Chinese medicine it is Liver Qi stagnation affecting the Spleen and Stomach, causing Qi to stagnate and rise in the Stomach Channel. You need to smooth Liver Qi, descend Stomach Qi, and calm the Mind. Treat points H7 and St18. Dispersing Liv3, LI4, and Sp6 may also be helpful.

Herbs *Agnus castus*
Oils *Chamomile, melissa, cypress*

H7 and St18

H7 is on the wrist crease on the little finger side of the palm. Calm it to calm the Mind and promote Blood circulation. Find St18 4 thumb widths from the mid line between the 5th and 6th ribs, below the nipple. Calm this point to reduce breast distension and help descend Stomach Qi.

Liv3
(page 25)

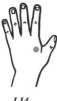

LI4
(page 24)

Sp6
(page 25)

MENOPAUSE

For some women this is a time of physical and emotional flux. Symptoms can include hot flashes, tiredness, irritability, insomnia, palpitations, vaginal irritation, and aching joints. Western medicine regards this as a natural process of cessation of menstruation at the end of reproductive life. In Chinese medicine it represents an imbalance in Kidney Qi, creating Yin Yang disharmony and leading to imblance of Qi and Blood in the Heart, Spleen, and Liver. You need to nourish Kidney Yin and eliminate Heat. Treat points K6 and H6. Tonifying CV6 may also be helpful.

Herbs *Motherwort, agnus castus, raspberry leaf, chamomile*
Oils *Cypress, chamomile, marigold*

H6
Find this point half a thumb width from the wrist crease on the forearm, on the little finger side of the palm. Disperse it to move Blood stagnation and Heat affecting the Heart, to help stop flushes and night sweats, and calm the Mind.

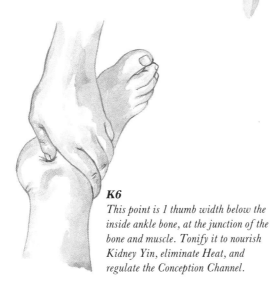

K6
This point is 1 thumb width below the inside ankle bone, at the junction of the bone and muscle. Tonify it to nourish Kidney Yin, eliminate Heat, and regulate the Conception Channel.

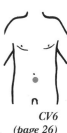

CV6
(page 26)

WEAK SEXUAL VITALITY

The pattern of sexual apathy, cold feelings inside, low back pain, poor memory, pale complexion, and poor appetite and digestion, often run together. Western and Chinese medicine regard this as a complex social, psychological problem, due to stress, emotional and nutritional factors, and the pressures of modern living. In Chinese medicine it is also a weakness of Kidney Yin and Yang Qi. You need to strengthen the Kidney. Treat points B47 and GV4. Tonifying B23, CV4, Sp6, and K6 may also be helpful.

CAUTION Never use Sp6 during pregnancy.

Herbs *American ginseng, red deer antler*
Oils *Melissa*

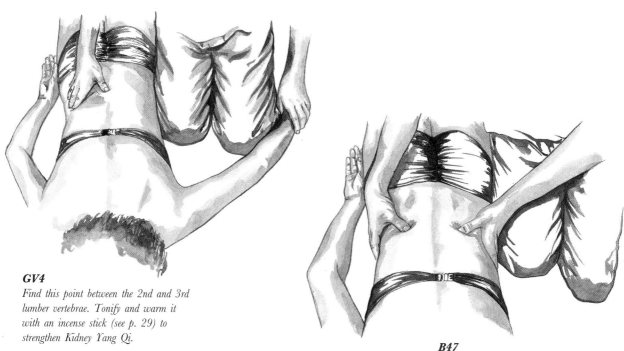

GV4
Find this point between the 2nd and 3rd lumber vertebrae. Tonify and warm it with an incense stick (see p. 29) to strengthen Kidney Yang Qi.

B47
These points are 4 finger widths either side of the spine, level with the 2nd and 3rd lumbar vertebrae. Tonify them and warm with your hand or a hotwater bottle. This strengthens the Kidneys and creates an inner feeling of sexual ease.

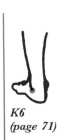

K6
(page 71)

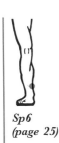

Sp6
(page 25)

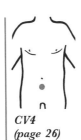

CV4
(page 26)

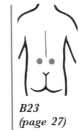

B23
(page 27)

Bones and joints

The stresses and tensions of modern living, and poor postural habits, take their toll on your skeleton over the years. You need daily exercise, a good diet, and plenty of relaxation and sleep to keep it healthy. Avoid overworking any part of your frame as this leads to imbalance. Acupressure can help relieve discomfort in the joints, whether produced by bad posture or injury. Remove Damp and Heat to reduce inflammation, move stagnant Blood away from the area, and move Qi and fresh Blood into it.

For how to use herbs and oils see age 30. For techniques for stimulating pressure points see page 29.

ARTHRITIS AND ACHING JOINTS

The joints may be inflamed - hot, swollen, red, and painful - or there may be only a vague aching, with gradual deterioration of the joint. According to Western medicine the causes of arthritis are injury, obesity, postural abnormality, infection, or wear and tear. In Chinese medicine the causes are weakness of the Kidneys and obstruction of Qi and Blood, and invasion of Wind, Cold, Damp, and Heat that lodge in the muscles and joints. Treat points GV14 and B11 . Tonifying K6, Sp6, GB39, TH6, and GB34 may also be helpful.

CAUTION Never use Sp6 during pregnancy.

Herbs *Guiacum, devil's claw, nettles, quince, meadowsweet, garlc. For inflammation use red clover and barberry.*
Oils *Marjoram*

CAUTION Never use marjoram oil or devil's claw during pregnancy.

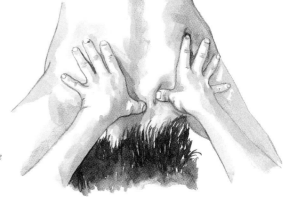

GV14 and B11

GV14 governs the Yang Channels. Find it between the 7th cervical and 1st thoracic vertebrae (left in illustration). Disperse it to clear Wind and Cold. The B11 points are 2 finger widths either side of the spine, level with the gap between the 1st and 2nd thoracic vertebrae (right in illustration). Disperse them to clear Wind. These are special points for the bones.

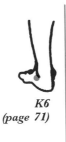

K6
(page 71)

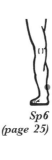

Sp6
(page 25)

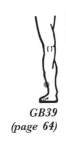

GB39
(page 64)

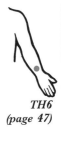

TH6
(page 47)

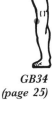

GB34
(page 25)

NECK AND SHOULDERS

The neck and shoulder joints are shallow and supported by interlacing ligaments and tendons, to allow a wide variety and range of movements. Short, sharp movements, or a whiplash or wrenching injury, can lead to damage of the soft tissue. Treat points SI12 and LI15. Dispersing GV14 and GB20, and tonifying LI4 may also be helpful.

CAUTION If the pain is severe or radiates down the arms, consult a doctor. Never use LI4 during pregnancy.

Herbs *Cinnamon stick, ginger root*
Oils *Chamomile, marigold, lavender*

CAUTION Never use marigold oil during pregnancy.

First aid for injuries

Apply an ice pack to the injured part for 20 minutes immediately, and then twice daily while pain and swelling persist, or apply a comfrey poultice or compress to the injured part. Hold it in place with an elastic bandage.

Elevate and support the part and move the joints gently in that position.

If the pain and swelling do not subside in 48 hours, or if there may be a fracture, seek professional help.

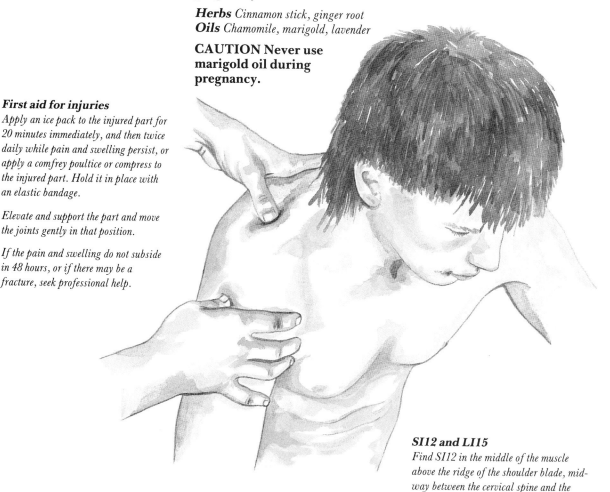

SI12 and LI15

Find SI12 in the middle of the muscle above the ridge of the shoulder blade, midway between the cervical spine and the tip of the shoulder. Disperse this point to move obstructions of Qi and Blood in the neck and shoulders. LI15 is on the outside of the shoulder, in the dimple created when the arm is raised to the side. Disperse it to move Qi and Blood.

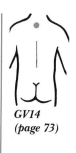

GV14
(page 73)

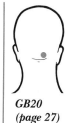

GB20
(page 27)

LI4
(page 24)

ELBOW

The elbow is a shallow joint, strongly supported by overlapping ligaments and tendons, with a large range of movement. Most injuries damage these ligaments and tendons and result from rapid jerking or small repetitive movements. Falls can lead to bone fractures. Treat points LI12, TH5, and LI11. Dispersing LI4 and LI10, and tonifying GB34 may also be helpful.

CAUTION Never use LI4 during pregnancy.

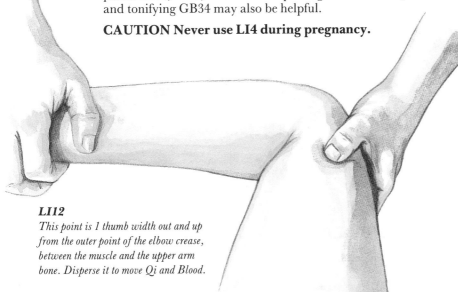

LI12

This point is 1 thumb width out and up from the outer point of the elbow crease, between the muscle and the upper arm bone. Disperse it to move Qi and Blood.

TH5 and LI11

Find TH5 2 thumb widths above the wrist crease in the middle of the back of the forearm. Disperse it to relax the tendons and remove blockages in the Yang Channels of the arm. LI11 is at the end of the outside crease of the elbow. Disperse it to move Qi and Blood and clear Heat in the Large Intestine Channel.

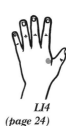

LI4
(page 24)

LI10
(page 64)

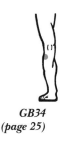

GB34
(page 25)

HAND AND WRIST

The hand and wrist joints are a complex system of levers and pulleys. They are strong and allow a wide range of movement.

When you fall you automatically put your hands out to save yourself, and this can lead to wrist injuries. There may be pain and swelling around the ligaments either side of the joint, or bone fracture. Treat points LI5, SI5, and TH4.

For hand pain or injuries treat points LI4 and SI3.

LI4 and SI3

LI4 is in the web between the thumb and index finger on the back of the hand. Disperse it to move Qi and Blood and dispel Wind. Find SI3 on the back of the hand between the bone and muscle, just before the knuckle of the little finger. Disperse it to move Qi and Blood, and remove stiffness in the spine.
CAUTION Never use LI4 during pregnancy.

LI5 and SI5

Find LI5 in the hollow at the base of the thumb on the side of the wrist joint. Disperse it to move Qi and Blood and clear Heat from the Large Intestine Channel. SI5 is in the hollow on the little finger side of the wrist joint. Disperse this point to move Qi and Blood, and clear Heat from the Small Intestine Channel.

TH4

This point is in the middle of the wrist joint on the back of the hand. Disperse it to move Qi and Blood and relax the tendons.

HIPS AND LUMBAR SPINE

The deep sockets in the hip joints allow maximum stability but only a narrow range of movement. The lumbar spine and pelvis consist of large bones with thick, strong ligament and muscular supports. Wear and tear and stiffness are very common, and often caused by bad lifting habits and posture. Treat points GB30 and B26. Tonifying B23, B54, and GB34 may also be helpful.

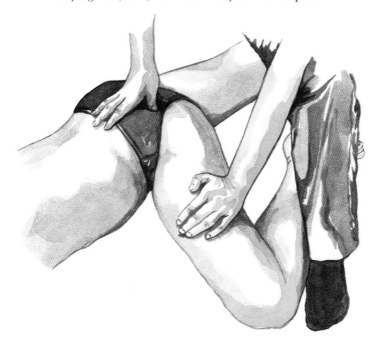

GB30

Find this point on the side of the buttock, two-thirds out along the line from the middle of the sacrum to the top of the thigh bone. Disperse it to move Qi and Blood obstruction in the pelvis and hip.

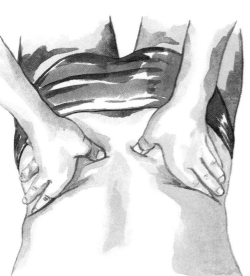

B26

These points are 2 finger widths either side of the spine, level with the 5th lumbar and 1st sacral vertebrae. Disperse them to move Qi and Blood, and strengthen the ligament that stabilizes the lumbar and sacral spine.

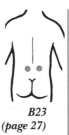

B23
(page 27)

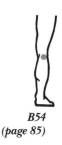

B54
(page 85)

GB34
(page 25)

KNEE

Your knees take a lot of your body weight but are not very stable. Twisting your foot while your weight is on it can lead to injuries in the cartilage and ligaments of the knee. There will be immediate pain and swelling, and the knee may "lock" so you cannot bend or straighten it.

KNEE PAIN ON BENDING

Treat points St35 and Xiyan. Dispersing GB34 may also be helpful.

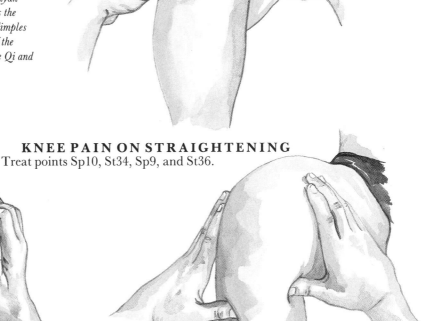

St35 and Xiyan

St35 (left in illustration) and Xiyan (right in illustration), known as the "eyes of the knee", are in the 2 dimples below the kneecap, either side of the ligament. Disperse them to move Qi and Blood and reduce pain.

KNEE PAIN ON STRAIGHTENING

Treat points Sp10, St34, Sp9, and St36.

Sp10 and St34

Sp10 (right in illustration) is 2 thumb widths above the top of the kneecap and 2 thumb widths toward the inside of the thigh. Disperse it to move Qi and to move and cool the Blood. Find St34 (left in illustration) 2 thumb widths above the top of the kneecap in line with its outside edge. Disperse this point to move Qi and Blood stagnation locally and in the Stomach Channel.

Sp9 and St36

Find Sp9 (right in illustration) on the inside of the leg below the knee joint, in the depression between the tibia and the calf muscle. Disperse it to move Qi and Blood, and remove Damp and Heat. St36 (left in illustration) is 4 finger widths below the tip of the kneecap outside the tibia. Disperse it to move and strengthen Qi and Blood, and remove Damp.

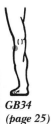

GB34
(page 25)

ANKLE

The ankle is designed to take all your weight and still be flexible. It is a strong joint when the foot is flexed, but it is easily twisted when the foot is pointed. This can cause ligament damage, with pain and swelling just under and around the ankle bones, or fracture. Treat points K3 and St41. Dispersing B60 and tonifying GB34 may also be helpful.

CAUTION Never use B60 during pregnancy.

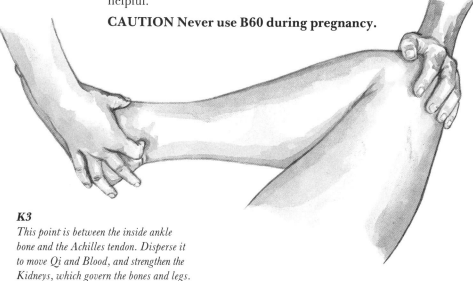

K3

This point is between the inside ankle bone and the Achilles tendon. Disperse it to move Qi and Blood, and strengthen the Kidneys, which govern the bones and legs.

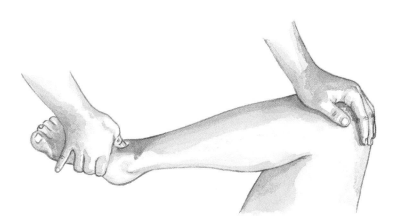

St41

Find St41 in the middle of the foot, in front of the ankle joint. Disperse it to move Qi and Blood and clear Heat from the Stomach Channel.

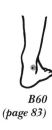

B60
(page 83)

GB34
(page 25)

Muscles

You need regular exercise, rest, and a balanced diet to keep your muscles strong and elastic. When a muscle is damaged, stagnation of Blood and Body Fluids causes swelling and pain. As the muscle heals the fibres tend to shorten, so it is less flexible, leading to stiffness and weakness. You need to remove Damp and Heat to reduce inflammation, move stagnant Blood away from the area, and move Qi and fresh Blood to replace it.

For how to use herbs and oils see page 30. For techniques for stimulating pressure points see page 29.

CAUTION If there is muscle wasting, that is the muscle is smaller than the corresponding muscle on the other side of the body, seek professional help.

STIFFNESS

When you start a new exercise programme it is easy to overdo the initial sessions. As you exercise, the blood supply to the muscles is increased, which in turn increases the tissue fluid around the muscle cells. The waste products from the cells and the tissue fluid cause stiffness. Stiffness may also be due to lack of exercise, ageing, or microscopic tears in the muscles, which occur during exercise.

You need to invigorate Qi and Blood circulation locally, and strengthen Qi and Blood generally. Treat points TH5 and GB34. Tonifying St36 and dispersing TH15 may also be helpful.

Herbs *Cayenne pepper linament, ginger, myrrh*
Oils *Lavender*

TH5
This point is 2 thumb widths above the wrist crease in the middle of the back of the forearm. Disperse it to regulate the surface Qi that nourishes the muscles and relaxes the tendons.

GB34
This is a special point for all muscle and tendon problems. Find it in the depression on the outside of the leg, below the knee joint and in front of and below the top of the fibula. Tonify this point to calm Liver Qi and remove Damp and Heat.

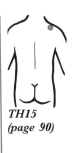

TH15
(page 90)

ST36
(page 25)

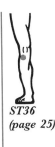

SHIATSU TECHNIQUES TO LOOSEN STIFF THIGHS AND CALVES

The aching, heaviness, and stiffness commonly felt after exercise are a result of accumulated waste products between the muscle fibres. Stretching the fibres at right angles to the direction they lie helps to squeeze these out.

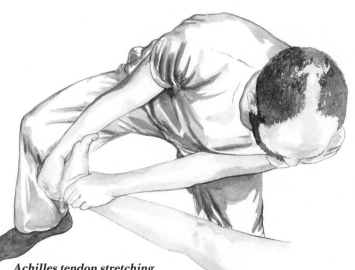

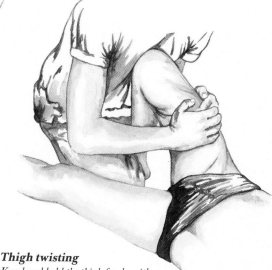

Achilles tendon stretching

Support the instep firmly with one hand and hold the heel with the other, so your forearm rests along the sole of the foot. Push firmly toward the body.

CAUTION Do not use this technique on hyper-extended knees (when the knees bend slightly the wrong way beyond the straight leg position).

Thigh twisting

Kneel and hold the thigh firmly with both hands, leaning your breastbone on the knee for support. Rotate the thigh muscles to the right and left 3 or 4 times.

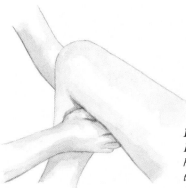

Pulling calf muscle

Either grasp the calf in both hands or hold the calf with one hand and support the knee with the other. Rotate the calf to the left and right 3 or 4 times.

BACKACHE

The vertebrae and the discs between them are like the upright pole in a tent, with the muscles on either side of them acting as guy ropes. Too much lifting, especially turning and lifting simultaneously, or bending, can cause backache. If you are prone to backache, it could be due to back weakness, which can be inherited, for example, due to height, or can result from injury. Poor posture and lack of exercise can compound back problems. Treat She Qi Zhui. Tonifying B23, B25, and GV4 can also be helpful.

CAUTION If the symptoms are severe seek professional guidance. Never apply pressure to She Qi Zhui if the pain extends down the legs.

Herbs Saw palmetto, nettles, devil's claw
Oils Black pepper, lavender

CAUTION Never use devil's claw in pregnancy.

She Qi Zhui
This point is in the middle of the spine between the 5th lumbar vertebra and the 1st sacral segment. Tonify and/or warm it with an incense stick (see p. 29), to strengthen the lower spine and reduce pain.
CAUTION Never apply pressure here if the pain extends down the legs. Seek professional help.

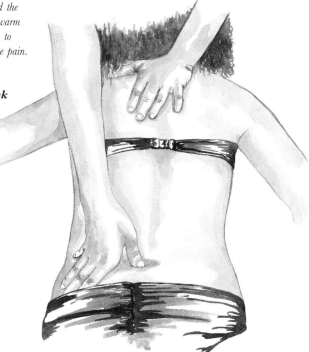

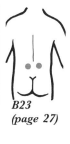

B23
(page 27)

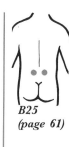

B25
(page 61)

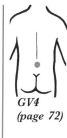

GV4
(page 72)

SCIATICA

If a disc is damaged the soft tissue around it swells and presses on the nerves. Pain then radiates down the back or side of the leg. Acupressure and herbal poultices will help relieve the pain. When sciatica is affecting the side of the leg, treat points GB30 and GB31. Dispersing GB34 and GB39 may also be helpful. For sciatica along the back of the leg, treat B57 (see p. 85) and B60. Dispersing B54, B26, and B23 may also be helpful.

CAUTION Sciatica may be due to disc problems, spinal arthritis, or even tumours. Seek professional guidance immediately.

Never use B60 during pregnancy.

FIRST AID TREATMENT

Rest, lying flat on your back on a hard surface. Do not lift, or stand for prolonged periods.

Herbs *Apply hypericum tincture and/or a comfrey poultice along the line of pain.*

Oils *Chamomile, geranium, lavender, marjoram*

CAUTION Never use marjoram oil during pregnancy.

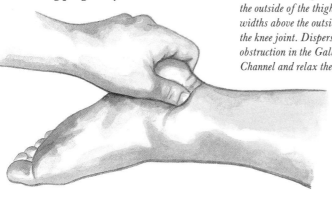

B60

Find this point on the outside of the ankle, halfway between the outside ankle bone and the Achilles tendon. Disperse it to reduce pain in the back by moving stagnant Qi and clearing Heat.

CAUTION Never use B60 during pregnancy.

GB30 and GB31

GB30 is on the side of the buttock, two-thirds out along the line from the middle of the sacrum to the top of the thigh bone. Disperse this point to move obstruction of Qi in the pelvis and hip and down the Gall Bladder Channel in the leg. Find GB31 on the outside of the thigh, 7 thumb widths above the outside crease of the knee joint. Disperse it to move obstruction in the Gall Bladder Channel and relax the tendons.

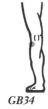

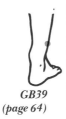

GB34
(page 84)

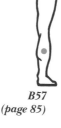

GB39
(page 64)

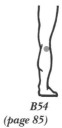

B57
(page 85)

B54
(page 85)

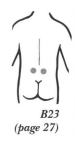

B26
(page 77)

B23
(page 27)

ACHING LEGS AND FEET

At the end of the day or after standing for prolonged periods the body becomes tired and the circulation sluggish. In both Chinese and Western medicine poor circulation leads to congestion, heaviness, and aching. You need to strengthen Qi and Blood and improve circulation in the legs and feet and the rest of the body. Treat points St36 and GB34, and disperse B57 (see opposite page).

Herbs *Foot bath: lavender, rosemary, ginger*
Oils *Lavender*

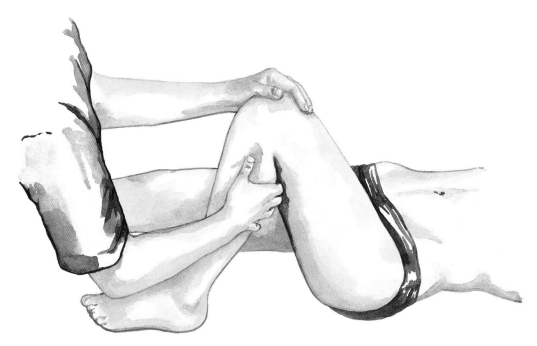

St36 and GB34

Find St36 4 finger widths below the top of the knee outside the tibia. Tonify and/ or warm this point with an incense stick (see p. 29) to promote the production and circulation of Qi and Blood, and strengthen the legs. GB34 regulates the contraction and relaxation of the muscles. It is in the depression on the outside of the leg, below the knee joint, in front of and below the top of the fibula. Tonify and/or warm this point with an incense stick (see p. 29).

MUSCLE CRAMP

Local spasms can be a result of fatigue during exercise or overwork. Many people get leg cramp at night, with severe pain and a hard, knotted feeling in the muscle. Western medicine explains this as fatigue or nervous system reflexes affecting blood circulation and the muscle. The Chinese view is that cramp arises from local stagnation and/or deficiency of Qi and Blood, so you need to regulate these. Treat points B57 and B54. Dispersing Liv3 and GB34 may also be helpful. For writer's cramp disperse LI4.

CAUTION Never use LI4 during pregnancy.

NOTE It is important to stretch the affected muscle to align the fibres, and to drink plenty of water, which carries vital tissue salts to the muscles.

Herbs *Quince, ginger, chamomile. Baths: lavender, rosemary*
Oils *Pine, cypress, marjoram*

CAUTION Never use marjoram oil during pregnancy.

B57
B57 is in the middle of the back of the calf where the muscle and tendon meet. Disperse this point, starting with a gentle "brushing" action and gradually working more deeply, to move Qi and Blood in the area.

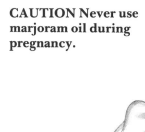

B54
Find this point in the middle of the crease on the back of the knee. Disperse it to improve circulation in the lower leg and remove Damp, which could have been the initial cause of the congestion.

Liv3
(page 25)

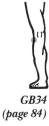
GB34
(page 84)

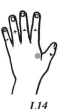
L14
(page 24)

Sense organs

Your eyes and ears are among the most delicate and complicated structures of your body. As well as enabling you to take in sights and sounds they are also essential for balance. The pressures of modern living, poor diet, and pollution, all "deaden" your senses, causing discomfort and leaving you less able to communicate with the world at large. Acupressure and herbs are useful for simple problems with the sense organs.

CAUTION If symptoms are severe, or come on suddenly, consult your doctor immediately.

For how to use herbs and oils see page 30. For techniques for stimulating pressure points see page 29.

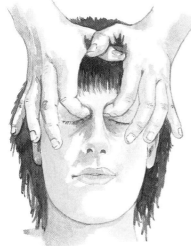

B1
Find this point just above the inner corner of the eye, between the side of the nose and the margin of the eye. Disperse it to eliminate Heat, improve Qi and Blood circulation, and nourish the Liver.

SORE EYES

Red, painful, sore, swollen, itching, and bloodshot eyes may be symptoms of sinusitis or a cold, or result from exposure to dust and wind. In Western medicine this is external irritation, strain, or inflammation due to infection. In Chinese medicine the Liver Blood nourishes the eyes and keeps them bright. Sore eyes arise from external Wind and Heat, or Liver disharmony, accompanied by irritability and anger. You need to clear Wind and Heat, and nourish the Liver. Treat points Tai Yang, B1, Liv2, and GB37. Dispersing GB20 and LI4 may also be helpful.

**CAUTION Since the eyes are very delicate, always consult your doctor about eye problems.
Never use LI4 during pregnancy.**

Herbs *Eyewash: eyebright; raspberry leaf; buckwheat leaves, strained thoroughly.*
Internally: chrysanthemum flowers; honeysuckle blossoms
Oils *Lavender*

Liv2 and GB37
Liv2 is on the top of the foot in the web between the 1st and 2nd toes. Disperse this point to clear Liver Heat and move stagnant Qi. Find GB37 5 thumb widths above the outside ankle bone in front of the fibula. Disperse it to reduce Liver and Gall Bladder Heat, thus brightening the eyes.

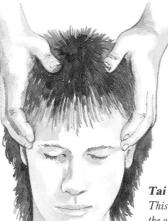

Tai Yang
This point is 1 thumb width away from the outside bony margin of the eye, level with the top of the ear. Disperse it to reduce Heat, swelling, and pain.

GB20
(page 27)

LI4
(page 25)

EARACHE

Symptoms include pain, headache, inflammation, discharge, dull hearing, and tinnitus (ringing in the ear). Western medicine sees most earache as arising from middle ear or external ear infections, though it may also be due to wax, boils, neuralgia, or eczema. In Chinese medicine sudden acute earache is often due to external Wind and Heat invading the ear, or rising toxic Heat in the Gall Bladder Channel. You need to clear the Wind, Heat, and toxins. Treat points TH3, TH17, and SI19. Dispersing GB20 and LI4 may also help.

CAUTION If pain is severe or there is a discharge or deafness, consult your doctor.
Never use LI4 during pregnancy.
Herbs *External use: mullein poultice; tincture of myrrh*
Oils *Lavender, add 1 drop to 1 tsp of warm olive oil, dip in cotton wool and place in ear.*

CAUTION Never use myrrh during pregnancy.

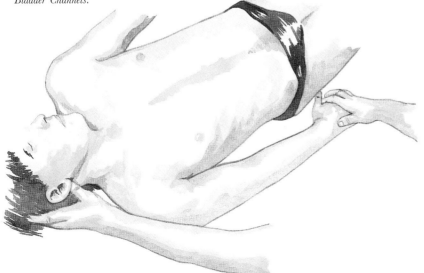

TH3 and TH17
TH3 is on the back of the hand in the furrow just before the 4th and 5th knuckles. Disperse this point to clear Heat, unblock the ears, and regulate Qi. Find TH17 in the small hollow behind the ear lobe, between the jaw and the skull. Disperse it to clear Wind and reduce Heat in the Liver and Gall Bladder Channels.

SI19
Find this point in the depression formed between the jaw joint and front of the middle of the ear, when the mouth is open. Disperse it to clear Wind and Heat and the Channels in and around the ear.

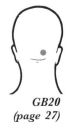

LI4
(page 25)

GB20
(page 27)

Summary of points

This summary lists all the points used in Part Two. They are listed by Channel, and the order of Channels follows the horary rhythm – the route of Qi in the body through the day (see p. 23). To locate a point, look at the treatment plan, this summary, and the Channels diagrams (pp. 22-23).

Major acupressure points
The following points are the 12 most commonly used in the treatments in this book. Refer to the illustrations on pages 24-27 for more help in locating them.
HP6, LI4, Sp6, GB34, St36, Liv3, CV4, CV6, GB20, B18, B20, B23.

LUNG

Lu1 *Below the bony prominence in front of the shoulder, under the shoulder end of the collar bone.*

Lu6 *7 thumb widths above the wrist crease on the inside of the forearm, in line with the thumb.*

Lu7 *2 finger widths above the wrist crease on the thumb side of the radius.*

Lu9 *On the thumb side of the wrist crease.*

Lu10 *2 finger widths down from the wrist crease, along the palm side of the thumb.*

Lu11 *On the outside corner of the thumbnail bed.*

LARGE INTESTINE

LI4 *On the back of the hand in the web between the thumb and index finger.*
Caution Never use this point during pregnancy. It can cause miscarriage.

LI5 *In the hollow at the base of the thumb on the side of the wrist joint.*

LI10 *2 thumb widths below the crease on the outside of the elbow, in line with the middle of the back of the wrist.*

LI11 *At the end of the outside crease of the elbow.*

LI12 *1 thumb width out and up from the outer point of the elbow crease, between the muscle and the upper arm bone.*

LI15 *In the dimple on the outside of the shoulder when the arm is raised sideways.*

LI20 *At the base of the nose, either side of the nostrils.*

STOMACH

St18 *In the space between the 5th and 6th ribs, in line with the nipple, 4 thumb widths from the mid line.*

St25 *2 thumb widths either side of the navel.*

St29 *2 thumb widths either side of the mid line and 4 thumb widths below the navel.*

St34 *2 thumb widths above the tip of the kneecap, in line with its outside edge.*

St35 *In the outside dimple of the knee joint below the kneecap, on the outside of the ligament.*

St36 *4 finger widths below the tip of the kneecap, outside the tibia.*

St37 *8 finger widths below the tip of the kneecap, outside the tibia.*

St41 *In the middle of the front of the ankle joint on the lower leg.*

St43 *On the top of the foot in the furrow between the 2nd and 3rd toes, where the two bones merge.*

St44 *On the top of the foot in the web at the root of the 2nd and 3rd toes.*

SPLEEN

Sp1 *On the outside corner of the nail bed of the big toe.*

Sp4 On the inside arch of the foot, just under the base of the long bone of the big toe.

Sp6 4 finger widths above the inside ankle bone, just behind the tibia. **Caution Never use this point during pregnancy. It can cause miscarriage.**

Sp8 4 finger widths below the inside of the knee joint between the calf muscle and the tibia.

Sp9 On the inside of the leg below the knee joint, in the depression between the tibia and the calf muscle.

Sp10 2 thumb widths above the tip of the kneecap and 2 thumb widths in, on the inside of the thigh.

HEART

H6 On the forearm half a thumb width up from the wrist crease, on the little finger side of the palm.

H7 On the wrist crease, on the little finger side.

SMALL INTESTINE

SI3 On the little finger side of the hand, between the bone and the muscle just before the knuckle and the little finger.

SI5 In the hollow on the little finger side of the wrist joint.

SI12 In the middle of the muscle above the ridge of the shoulder blade, halfway between the cervical spine and the tip of the shoulder.

SI19 In the depression formed when the mouth is open, between the jaw joint and the front of the middle part of the ear.

BLADDER

B1 Just above the inner corner of the eye, between the side of the nose and the margin of the eye.

B11 2 finger widths either side of the spine, level with the 1st and 2nd thoracic vertebrae.

B13 2 finger widths either side of the spine, level with the 3rd and 4th thoracic vertebrae.

B15 2 finger widths either side of the spine, between the lower borders of the shoulder blades, level with the 5th and 6th thoracic vertebrae.

B18 2 finger widths either side of the spine, level with the 9th and 10th thoracic vertebrae.

B20 2 finger widths either side of the spine, level with the 11th and 12th thoracic vertebrae.

B22 2 finger widths either side of the spine, level with the 1st and 2nd lumbar vertebrae.

B23 2 finger widths either side of the spine, level with the 2nd and 3rd lumbar vertebrae.

B25 2 finger widths either side of the spine, level with the 4th and 5th lumbar vertebrae.

B26 2 finger widths either side of the spine, at the level of the 5th lumbar vertebra and 1st sacral segment.

B32 in the 2nd sacral holes, either side of the sacral spine.

B47 4 finger widths either side of the spine, level with the 2nd and 3rd lumbar vertebrae, outside B23.

B54 In the middle of the crease on the back of the knee.

B57 In the middle of the back of the calf at the junction of the muscle and tendon.

B60 On the outside of the ankle between the ankle bone and the Achilles tendon. **Caution Never use this point during pregnancy. It can cause miscarriage.**

KIDNEY

K1 In the crease in the middle of the ball of the foot, at the colour change between the ball and sole.

K3 Inside the ankle between the inside ankle bone and the Achilles tendon.

K6 1 thumb width below the inside ankle bone, at the junction of the bone and muscle.

HEART PROTECTOR

HP6 2 thumb widths up from the palm side of the wrist crease, in the middle of the lower forearm.

TRIPLE HEATER

TH3 On the back of the hand in the furrow just before the 4th and 5th knuckles.

TH4 In the middle of the wrist joint on the back of the hand.

TH5 *2 thumb widths above the wrist crease in the middle of the back of the forearm.*

TH6 *4 finger widths above the wrist on the back of the forearm.*

TH15 *Above the ridge of the shoulder blade, just down from the highest point of the trapezius neck muscle, midway between the cervical spine and the tip of the shoulder.*

TH17 *In the small hollow behind the ear lobe between the jaw, skull, and ear.*

GALL BLADDER

GB20 *At the base of the skull in the hollow in the hairline, between the front and back neck muscles behind the bony prominence behind the ear.*

GB30 *On the side of the buttock, two-thirds out along a line from the middle of the sacrum to the top of the thigh bone.*

GB31 *On the outside of the thigh, 7 thumb widths above the outside crease of the knee joint.*

GB34 *In the depression on the outside of the lower leg, below the knee joint, in front of and below the top of the fibula.*

GB37 *5 thumb widths above the outside ankle bone in front of the fibula.*

GB39 *4 finger widths above the outside ankle bone on the side of the lower leg, in front of the fibula.*

GB41 *On the top of the foot in the furrow between the 4th and 5th toes, outside the tendon of the little toe.*

LIVER

Liv1 *On the inside corner of the nail bed of the big toe.*

Liv2 *On the top of the foot in the web between the 1st and 2nd toes.*

Liv3 *On the top of the foot in the furrow between the 1st and 2nd toes, where the bones merge.*

Liv13 *Below the free end of the 11th rib, at the bottom and side of the rib cage.*

CONCEPTION VESSEL

CV3 *4 thumb widths below the navel, on the mid line of the belly.*

CV4 *4 finger widths below the navel, on the mid line of the belly.*

CV6 *2 finger widths below the navel, on the mid line of the belly.*

CV12 *4 thumb widths above the navel, on the mid line of the belly.*

CV14 *8 finger widths above the navel, on the mid line of the belly.*

CV17 *On the breastbone, midway between the nipples.*

GOVERNING VESSEL

GV1 *At the very end of the spine on the mid line, halfway between the coccyx and the anus.*

GV4 *On the mid line of the spine between the 2nd and 3rd lumbar vertebrae.*

GV14 *On the back of the neck between the 7th cervical and 1st thoracic vertebrae.*

GV20 *In the middle of the top of the head, halfway between the ears.*

GV26 *In the middle of the furrow between the upper lip and the nose.*

POINTS NOT ON THE CHANNELS

Yintang *In the middle of the forehead between the eyebrows, just above the nose.*

Bitong *In the small hollow on the side of the bridge of the nose.*

Tai Yang *1 thumb width behind the bony margin of the eye, on a line from the eye to the top of the ear.*

Ding Chuan *A half thumb width either side of GV14, which is between the 7th cervical and 1st thoracic.*

Xiyan *The inside dimple of the knee joint below the kneecap, either side of the ligament.*

She Qi Zhi Xia *Between the 5th lumbar vertebra and 1st sacral segment, in the middle of the spine.*

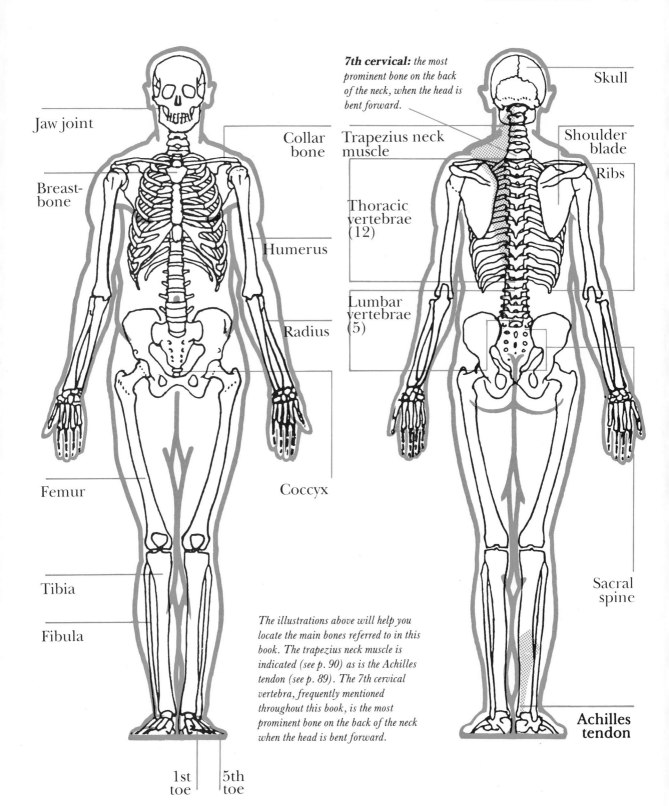

Jaw joint

Breast-bone

Femur

Tibia

Fibula

1st toe

5th toe

Collar bone

Humerus

Radius

Coccyx

7th cervical: *the most prominent bone on the back of the neck, when the head is bent forward.*

Trapezius neck muscle

Thoracic vertebrae (12)

Lumbar vertebrae (5)

Skull

Shoulder blade

Ribs

Sacral spine

Achilles tendon

The illustrations above will help you locate the main bones referred to in this book. The trapezius neck muscle is indicated (see p. 90) as is the Achilles tendon (see p. 89). The 7th cervical vertebra, frequently mentioned throughout this book, is the most prominent bone on the back of the neck when the head is bent forward.

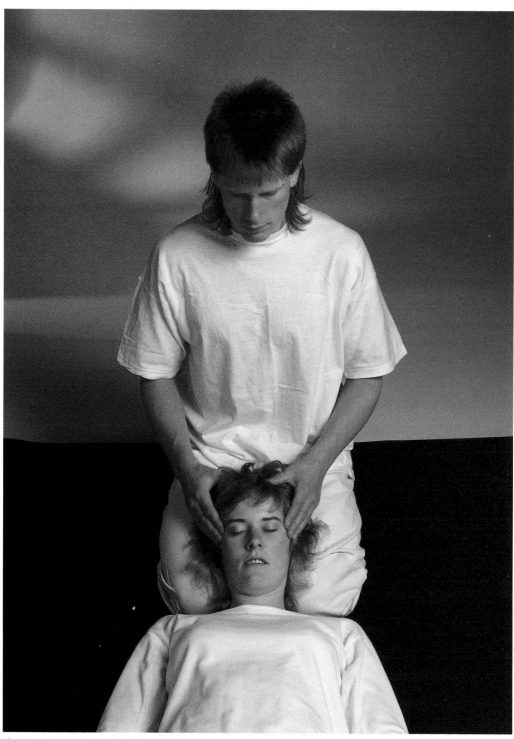

Calming the Tai Yang points alleviates a headache.

Index

Bold type indicates main entry; *italics* indicate illustrations.

A

abdominal pain 19, 58, 60
Achilles tendon 81
aching feet **84**
aching joints 71, 73
aching legs **84**
acidic stomach **59**
acupressure
    how acupressure works 8
    safety of treatment 11
    self-treatment 11
    treatment techniques 28–9
agnus castus 70, 71
agrimony 69
AIDS 9
alcoholism 9
alfalfa 58
allergies 9
American ginseng 38, 72
anaemia 25
aniseed 60
ankle **79**
anxiety 9, 24, 25, **42**, 45
apathy 44, 46
    sexual **72**
appetite loss 19, 44, 57, 72
arthritis **73**
asthma **54**

B

B1 *22*, *86*, 89
B11 *22*, *73*, 89
B13 *22*, *46*, 48, 54, *55*, 89
B15 *22*, *44*, 89
B18 *22*, *27*, 61, *68*, 89
B20 *22*, *27*, *46*, *57*, *62*, *68*, 89
B22 *22*, *62*, 89
B23 *22*, *27*, *46*, 54, *57*, *62*, 67, *68*, 72, 77,
    82, 83, 89
B25 *22*, *61*, 62, 82, 89
B26 *22*, 77, 83, 89
B32 *22*, *63*, 89
B47 *22*, *72*, 89
B54 *22*, 63, 77, 83, *85*, 89
B57 *22*, *65*, 83, 84, *85*, 89
B60 *22*, *23*, 63, 79, *83*, 89
Bach Flower Remedy 45
back problems 72, **82** *see also* spine
barberry 73
basil 61
basil oil 52
baths 31
bayberry 65
bed-wetting 18
belching 58
bergamot oil 42, 44, 57, 59
Bitong *22*, *23*, *52*, 90
black pepper oil 50, 64, 82
black sesame seeds 61
Bladder 35
Bladder Channel 21, *22*, *23*, 35 *for points
    on this Channel see* B
bladder infection 63
blisters 11
bloating 58, **60**, 66, 70

Blood 25, 26, 27
blood pressure 9
    high 9, 11, 65
    low 11, 65
blurred vision 45
boils 11
bones **73**
bowel 24
breasts 66, 70
breathing 10
breathlessness 19
bronchitis **55**
buckwheat leaves 86
burdock 51

C

calf muscles 81
calming *29*
cancer 9
caraway 58, 66
cardamom 57, 60
cartilage, knee 78
catnip 60
cayenne pepper liniment 80
cayenne pepper tincture 39, 45
chamomile 41, 42, 59, 71, 85
chamomile oil 40, 41, 44, 57, 59, 62, 70,
    71, 74, 83
Channel-opening techniques 10, 32–5
Channels 8, 14, 20–21, *22–23*
cherry bark 55
Chi *see* Qi
chrysanthemum flowers 86
cinnamon 50, 57, 62, 64
cinnamon stick 74
circulation 9, 25, 27, 64
cleavers 63
clothing 9, 28
clover 73
clover blossom 41, 42
cold extremities **64**
colds 24, 27, **50**
comfrey 83
comfrey root 65
complexion 13, 38, 72
compresses 31
Conception Vessel Channel *22*, *23*, 26
    for points on this Channel see CV
congestion 24, 27, 51, 52
consciousness, loss of 45
constipation **61**
coriander 60
corn silk 63
couchgrass 63
coughing 19
cramp **85**
cumin 60
CV3 *22*, *23*, *63*, 66, 90
CV4 *22*, *23*, *26*, *38*, 39, 62, 67, 68, *69*, 72,
    90
CV6 *22*, *26*, *45*, 48, 56, *66*, 67, 71, 90
CV12 *22*, *42*, *58*, 60, 90
CV14 *22*, *23*, *42*, *44*, 90
CV17 *22*, *23*, *55*, 56, 90
cypress oil 62, 65, 66, 69, 70, 71, 85
cystitis **63**

D

dandelion and burdock 51
dandelion root 61, 63
deafness 87
dehydration 62
depression 18, 19, 38, **44,** 66, 70
devil's claw 73, 82
diabetes 9
diagnosis 13
diarrhoea 18, 19, **62**
digestion 14, 18, 19, 25, 57, 72
dill 59, 60
Ding Chuan *22*, *54*, 90
disc problems 83
disharmony 13, 15
dispersing *29*
dizziness 18, 19, 39, 45, 47, 68
dock 65
drug abuse 9
dry mouth 18, 19

E

earache **87**
echinacea 46, 55
elbow **75**
elderflower 51
elecampane root 54, 55
elimination **61**
emotions 18–19
Energy *see* Qi
eyebright 86
eyes, sore **86**
eyewash 86

F

fainting **39**
fatigue **38,** 44
    chronic **47**
feet, aching **84**
fennel 57, 60
fever 50, 51
first aid
    fainting 39
    injuries to bones and joints 74
    sciatica 83
flatulence **60**
flu *see* influenza
food 10
forehead headaches 40

G

Gall Bladder Channel 14, 21, *22*, *23*,
    25, 35 *for points on this Channel see* GB
garlic 64, 73
GB20 *22*, *23*, *27*, 40, 50, 51, 52, 74, 86,
    87, 90
GB30 *23*, 77, *83*, 90
GB31 *23*, *83*, 90
GB34 *23*, *25*, 73, 75, 77, 79, *80*, 83, *84*,
    85, 90
GB37 *23*, *86*, 90

GB39 *23, 64*, 73, 83, 90
GB41 *23, 47*, 90
geranium oil 69, 83
ginger 58, 64, 80, 84, 85
ginger and cinnamon twig tea 50
ginger oil 54
ginger root 63, 66, 74
ginseng 38, 72
Governing Vessel Channel *22, 23 for points on this Channel see* GV
guiacum 73
GV1 *22*, 65, 90
GV4 *22, 38*, 57, *72*, 82, 90
GV14 *22, 47, 50, 73*, 74, 90
GV20 *22*, 39, *41*, 65, 90
GV26 *22, 39*, 45, 90

H

H6 *22, 23, 71*, 89
H7 *22, 23*, 42, 44, *70, 89*
haemorrhoids **65**
hand **76**
hawthorn berries 62
headaches 11, 18, 19, 24, 25, 27, **40,** 47, 50, 51, 87
hearing loss 87
Heart 18, 19
Heart Channel 21, *22, 23*, 32 *for points on this Channel see* H
heartburn 59
heart disease 9
Heart Protector Channel 21, *22, 23*, 32 *for points on this Channel see* HP
heavy menstruation 67, **69**
herbs **30–1**
high blood presssure 9, 65
hips **77**
honey 53
honeysuckle blossoms 86
horary rhythm 23, 88
hot flushes 71
HP6 *22, 23*, 24, *42*, 44, 45, 58, 60, 64, 89
Huang Qi 46
huckleberry 62
huckleberry oil 62
hypericum tincture 83

I

immune system 9, **46**
incense sticks *29*
incontinence 15
indigestion **58**
influenza 51
   recurrent **48**
inhalation 31
insomnia 18, 19, 25, **44,** 46, 71
irritability 25, 60, 66, 70, 71

J

jasmine oil 44, 72
joint pains 19, 50, 71, 73

K

K1 *23, 45*, 89
K3 *23, 79*, 89
K6 *23, 71*, 72, 73, 89

Ki *see* Qi
Kidney 14, 15, 18, 19, 27, 34
Kidney Channel 21, *22, 23*, 25, 26, 34
   for points on this Channel see K
knee **78**

L

labour 25
Lao Tzu 16
Large Intestine Channel 14, 21, *22, 23*, 33 *for points on this Channel see* LI
lavender 44, 84, 85
lavender oil 38, 40, 42, 48, 51, 52, 54, 55, 58, 62, 74, 80, 82, 83, 84, 86
legs, aching 25, **84**
lemon balm 60
lemon grass oil 82
lemon oil 51, 64
lethargy 15, 47
LI4 *22, 23*, 24, 38, *41*, 46, 48, 50, 51, 52, 53, 54, 64, 70, 74, 75, *76*, 85, 86, 87, 88
LI5 *22, 23, 76*, 88
LI10 *22, 23, 64*, 75, 88
LI11 *22, 23, 51*, 75, 88
LI12 *22, 23*, 75, 88
LI15 *22, 23*, 74, 88
LI20 *22, 23*, 52, 88
Ling Zhi 46
Liv1 *22*, 69, 90
Liv2 *22, 86*, 90
Liv3 *22*, 25, *40, 41, 60*, 64, *66*, 69, 70, 85, 90
Liv13 *22, 58*, 90
Liver 18, 27
Liver Channel 14, 19, 21, *22, 23*, 25, 26, 34 *for points on this Channel see* Liv
low blood pressure 45
Lu1 *22, 23, 55*, 88
Lu6 *22, 23, 54*, 88
Lu7 *22, 23, 48, 50*, 88
Lu9 *22, 23, 55*, 88
Lu10 *22, 23, 51*, 88
Lu11 *22, 23, 53*, 88
lumbar spine **77**
Lung Channel *21, 22, 23, 33 for points on this Channel see* Lu
Lungs 19
lungwort 55

M

madder root 69
marigold oil 65, 71, 74
marjoram 60
marjoram oil 40, 42, 73, 83, 85
marshmallow 52, 63
marshmallow root 48
massage 31
meadowsweet 57, 73
melissa oil 45, 66, 70, 72
memory loss 72
menopause **71**
menstrual pain 25, **66, 67**
menstruation 19, 26
   heavy **69**
Meridians 8, 20
migraine headaches 19, 25, 40
miscarriage 11, 24, 30
motherwort 41, 42, 71

mouth ulcers 18
mullein 48, 55, 87
muscle cramp **85**
muscles 25, 80
myrrh 80
myrrh oil 65
myrrh, tincture of 87

N

nasal passages, congested 51, 52
nausea 24, 45, **58,** 59, 70
neck **74**
   stiffness 19, 50
neroli oil 41
nervous stomach 42
nervous system 9, **40**
nettles 54, 62, 63, 65, 73, 82
night sweating 18, 19
nose, runny 19, 52
numbness 39

O

obesity 9
oedema 15
oils 11, **30–1**
organ functions 14
Oriental medicine 9, 13, 16, 18

P

pain 47 *see also* abdominal pain, joint pains, period pain
   legs 25
   upper body 24
palpitations 18, 19, 44, 68, 71
panic attacks 42
passiflora 44
pattern of disharmony 13, 15
peppermint 40, 51, 58, 60
period pain 25, **66, 67**
piles **65**
pilewort 65
pine oil 48, 52, 54, 55, 85
pollution 18
post menstrual pain **68**
post viral syndrome **47**
poultices 31
pre-menstrual pain **66**
pre-menstrual tension **70**
pressure points 8, 10, 14, 20–7, 88–91
prickly ash bark 62
purgatives 61

Q

Qi 8, 10, 11, 14, 15, 16, 20, 29
quince 73, 85

R

raspberry leaf 62, 69, 71, 86
red clover 73
red deer antler 72
regurgitation 59
reproductive system **66**
reactions to treatment 11

respiration **50**
  shiatsu and acupressure techniques 56
restlessness 18, 19, 60
rib pressing 56
rosehips 62
rosemary 44, 84, 85
rosemary oil 54, 60, 61, 62, 73, 80, 82, 84
rue 87
runny nose 19, 52

S

safety 11
sandalwood oil 44
saw palmetto 55, 63, 82
scanty menstrual flow 68
scar tissue 11
sciatica **83**
self-treatment 11
sense organs **86**
sesame seeds 61
sexual apathy **72**
She Qi Zhi Xia *22, 82*, 90
shepherd's purse, tincture of 69
shiatsu techniques 56, 81
shock 19, **45**
shortness of breath 44
shoulders **74**
SI3 *22, 76*, 89
SI5 *22, 76*, 89
SI12 *22, 74*, 89
SI19 *23, 87*, 89
sinusitis 24, 27, **52**
skin rashes 11
sleeplessness 18, 19, 25, 44, 46, 71
Small Intestine Channel 21, *22, 23*, 33
  for points on this Channel see SI
smelling salts 30, 39
sneezing 19
sore throat **53**
Sp1 *23, 69*, 88
Sp4 *23, 60*, 89
Sp6 *23, 24, 25, 38, 39, 42, 44*, 55, 57, 64, 67, 70, 72, 73, 89
Sp8 *23, 66*, 89
Sp9 *23, 62, 78, 89*
Sp10 *23, 78*, 89
spine, lumbar **77**
Spleen 14, 18, 19, 25, 27
Spleen Channel 21, *22, 23*, 26, 34 *for points on this Channel see* Sp
squaw vine 69
St18 *22, 23, 70*, 88
St25 *22, 23*, 57, *58*, 61, 62, 88
St29 *22, 23, 63*, 88
St34 *22, 23, 78*, 88
St35 *22, 23, 78*, 88
St36 *22, 23, 25, 38, 39, 40, 42*, 45, 46, 55, 57, 58, 60, 62, 64, 67, 68, *78, 84*, 88
St37 *22, 23, 62*, 88
St41 *22, 23, 79*, 88
St43 *22, 23, 59*, 88
St44 *22, 23, 59*, 88
Star of Bethlehem 45
sterility 25
stiff neck 19, 50
stiffness 80, 81
Stomach 24, 25
stomach acidity **59**
Stomach Channel 14, 21, *22, 23*, 35 *for points on this Channel see* St
stomach, nervous 42

stress 9, **41**
sweating 19, 51
swollen breasts 66, 70

T

Tai Yang *23, 86*, 90
Taoism 16
teas 31
tension 27, **41**
TH3 *22, 87*, 89
TH4 *23, 76*, 89
TH5 *22, 23, 48, 75, 80*, 90
TH6 *22, 23, 47*, 61, 73, 90
TH15 *22*, 80, 90
TH17 *22, 87*, 90
thighs 81
thirst 18, 19, 51
throat, sore **53**
thyme 54
tinnitus 18, 19, 87
tiredness 19, 38, 46, 71
toxins 11
tonifying *29*
toothache 24
travel sickness 24
treatment plan 9, 15
Triple Heater Channel 21, *22, 23*, 33 *for points on this Channel see* TH

U

unconsciousness 45
Universal Qi 8, 10, 11
urine 13, 19

V

vaginal discharge 19
vaginal irritation 71
varicose veins 11
vision, blurred 45
vitality 9, **38**
  sexual **72**
voice 13
voice, weakness of 38
vomiting 18, 19, 45, 58

W

wave rocking 61
weather 18, 19
Western medicine 13
wild cherry bark 55
wild yam 66
wood betony 57
worry 9, 19, **42**
wounds 11
wrist **76**

X

Xiyan *22, 78*, 90

Y

yam 66
yarrow 65
yellow dock 65
Yin and Yang 14–15, 16–17
Yintang *22, 40*, 52, 90

Acknowledgements

Gaia Books would like to thank: Janine Christley, Eliza Dunlop, Lesley Gilbert, Libby Hoseason, Sarah Jarvis, Alison Jones, Sara Mathews, Susan Walby, and Mary Warren, for editorial and production work; Yvonne Dixon for the index; Mark Jarvis for additional photography (p. 19); Protocol Design Associates and Studio 21 for additional typesetting; Zoë Billingham, Juliet Hacking, Susan Henssen, Chris Jarmey, Debbie Jarmey, Gordon Lines, Callum Linton, Dave Thorp, and John Tindall for modelling; Vicki Pitman for advice on herbs; Barbara Blanchard, Dr Richard Donze, Lucy Lidell, and Roger Newman Turner for helpful comments and advice.

Bibliography

Kaptchuk, Ted J., 1983, *Chinese Medicine: The Web that has no Weaver*, Rider

Lidell, Lucinda, 1984, *The Book of Massage*, Ebury Press (UK), Simon & Schuster (US)

Mabey, Richard, 1988, *The Complete New Herbal*, Elm Tree Books (UK). Also published as *The New Age Herbalist*, Macmillan (US)

Maciocia, Giovanni, 1989, *The Foundations of Chinese Medicine*, Churchill Livingstone

O'Connor, John and Bensky, Dan, 1974, *Acupuncture – a comprehensive text*, Eastland Press, Seattle

Thie, John, 1979, *Touch for Health Manual*, De Vorss & Co

Thomas, Sara, 1989, *Massage for Common Ailments*, Sidgwick & Jackson (UK), Simon & Schuster (US), Angus&Robertson/HarperCollins (Aus)

Resources

The Shiatsu Society
Interchange Studios
Dalby Street
London NW5 3NQ
Tel: 0171 813 7772
Fax: 0171 813 7773

The European Shiatsu School
Central Administration
Highbanks
Lockeridge
Marlborough
Wilts SN8 4EQ

Australian Natural Therapists' Association Ltd
Suite 1, 2nd Floor
468-472 George Street
(P O Box A964)
Sydney NSW 2000

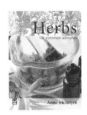

Herbs for Common Ailments

Anne McIntyre

ISBN 1 85675 055 8   **£8.99**

*Sets reliable, traditional knowledge in a modern context. It shows you how to use herbs for self help, prevention and cure; as well as the basics of herbalism and how to prepare your own herbs for safe treatments.

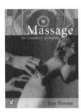

Massage for Common Ailments

Sara Thomas

ISBN 1 85675 031 0   **£8.99**

Transforms the ancient art of touch into a precise healing skill. With step-by-step illustrations, it demonstrates the strokes that soothe and heal, then applies them to specific ailments.

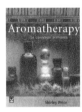

Aromatherapy for Common Ailments

Shirley Price

ISBN 1 85675 005 1   **£8.99**

Best-selling author Shirley Price provides an invaluable guide to the use of oils and treating a wide range of ailments. Includes a full-body aromatherapy massage routine.

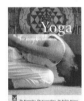

Yoga for Common Ailments

Dr R Monro, Dr Nagarathna and Dr Nagendra

ISBN 1 85675 010 8   **£8.99**

Simple sequences of yoga postures teach you how to counteract common disorders and enables you to design a programme for your personal needs.

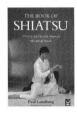

The Book of Shiatsu

Paul Lundberg

ISBN 1 85675 060 4   **£11.99**

A complete guide for the beginner and an excellent course book for students. Hands-on diagnosis is followed by a complete shiatsu massage.

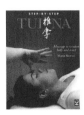

Step-by-Step Tui Na

Maria Mercati

ISBN 1 85675 038 8   **£14.99 hardback**
ISBN 1 85675 044 2   **£11.99 paperback**

Powerful, robust, energising massage for the treatment of chronic pain and to boost health and vitality.

To request a full catalogue of titles published by Gaia Books please call 01453 752985, fax 01453 752987 or write to Gaia Books Ltd., 20 High Street, Stroud, Gloucestershire, GL5 1AZ
e-mail address: sales@gaiabooks.co.uk   Internet address: http://www.gaiabooks.co.uk